This textbook has been published with t̠ ̠ ̠
support of WR Berkley Insurance (Europe) Ltd,
Heritage Direct Insurance Ltd, and Howden Medical
Insurance Services as an educational service for policyholders.
Their support and encouragement are very much appreciated.

Paul Lambden

THE OSTEOPATH'S GUIDE TO KEEPING OUT OF TROUBLE

A toolkit to help meet professional obligations
and avoid pitfalls in practice

Paul Lambden

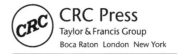

CRC Press
Taylor & Francis Group
Boca Raton London New York

CRC Press is an imprint of the
Taylor & Francis Group, an **informa** business

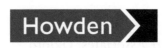

Radcliffe Publishing Ltd
18 Marcham Road
Abingdon
Oxon OX14 1AA
United Kingdom

www.radcliffe-oxford.com
Electronic catalogue and worldwide online ordering facility.

British Library Cataloguing in Publication Data

A catalogue record for this book is available from the British Library.

ISBN 1 85775 737 8

Typeset by Anne Joshua & Associates, Oxford

CONTENTS

PREFACE

Clinical practice has undergone a huge change over the last 30 years. It all used to be so simple. The patient would come to the surgery and explain to the osteopath the nature of the problem. The osteopath would examine the patient and notify the patient of what he (or occasionally she) had found. Treatment would then be prescribed and the necessary work undertaken. Patients would be unquestioning and grateful for whatever therapy they received. If the osteopath had an urge to explain in some detail to the patient what approach was anticipated, the patient would more than likely have waved the explanation away with a cheery, 'whatever you think, doc'. The osteopath would jot down a few, probably illegible, notes.

How different it all is now. We work in a litigious environment where adverse outcomes are viewed seriously. Osteopaths must be sure that they take careful histories, examine according to best practice, explain in sufficient detail the problem to be able to obtain valid consent, treat the patient with care and write notes that are sufficiently full and legible to ensure that the osteopath has a defence if a patient tries to take him (or her) to court.

It is probable that the treatment of today is of a much higher quality than a generation ago, but we have all paid a price to get it. Clinical work is now generally a much more stressful activity than it was in the past. The advent of risk management has hopefully started to reduce the risk of anything going wrong during clinical work and this book is an attempt to identify some of those areas where relatively simple changes may keep you safe, and where a bit of knowledge of the law and some simple ethical principles may support you in difficult times.

I have tried to keep the text relatively light and to avoid excessive detail. I have written it from the perspective of a medico-legal adviser. The availability of a trained medico-legal adviser at the other end of a telephone when a problem arises is often invaluable. The adviser can act as friend, adviser, supporter, confidant(e) and ally and his or her experience can often get an osteopath out of trouble quickly and efficiently.

Howden Insurance Services, for which I work, has recognised the huge value of effective medico-legal advice in times of trouble. Howden provides a high-quality insurance policy and it is a privilege to work with an organisation committed to excellence.

If you have any questions or nice comments about this book, please e-mail me at <u>paullambden@compuserve.com</u> – if you have any rude comments please keep them to yourself, because I am easily wounded.

Enjoy the book.

Paul Lambden
March 2005

ABOUT THE AUTHOR

Dr Paul Lambden BSc MB BS BDS FDSRCSEng MRCS(Eng) LRCP(Lond) DRCOG MHSM graduated in Medicine, Dentistry and Science at Guy's Hospital, London. After working initially in Oral Surgery and obtaining his Fellowship of the Royal College of Surgeons of England, he entered general medical and general dental practice, continuing the two for over 15 years. He was also a clinical tutor at St Bartholomew's Hospital, London.

In 1992 he left general practice to become the Chief Executive of East Hertfordshire NHS Trust, a whole district trust providing services for 300 000 people with a budget of over £65 million. He was also appointed a specialist adviser to the all-party Parliamentary Health Select Committee, which post he fulfilled for three years. In the late 1990s he became the Medical and Dental Principal of The St Paul International Insurance Company when it launched its professional indemnity (medical defence) programme for doctors and dentists. More recently he has worked as managing director of MIA General Insurance and is currently working at Howden Medical Insurance Services. He has recently been appointed Lecturer in Law and Ethics at the Kigezi International School of Medicine at Cambridge.

Paul is a regular writer on healthcare, management and medical defence topics. He has made a number of programmes for medical television channels and has been the author or co-author of half a dozen textbooks, including such subjects as the internet, law and ethics, the Human Rights Act and risk management in medicine and dentistry, and contributor to several more. He is a *Star Trek* fan.

DEDICATION

To Roy Lilley, my colleague and friend, with whom it has been my pleasure and privilege to write a number of books over recent years. He has taught me more about writing and communication than anyone else.

ACKNOWLEDGEMENTS

I am most grateful to Vincent Cullen, Head of Development at the General Osteopathic Council, to Charles Hunt, Vice Principal at the British School of Osteopathy, and to Paula Fletcher, Principal at the European School of Osteopathy, for their invaluable contributions, their peer review and proof-reading skills. The views expressed in the book are not necessarily theirs and they have given generously of their advice in a personal capacity only. Also my thanks to Elizabeth Blanchfield of Howden Insurance for her considerable assistance with the Health and Safety sections, and to Asgar Hassanali, also of Howden Insurance, for his advice on some of the sections.

Insurance to protect and support osteopaths in circumstances where they are accused of negligence, poor practice or inappropriate conduct is referred to as **'professional indemnity'** throughout the book. The old term, 'medical malpractice', is now in my view considered obsolete, if only because of the insulting implication that the practitioner must have done something wrong. It should be consigned to history.

THE OSTEOPATH'S GUIDE TO KEEPING OUT OF TROUBLE

THE OSTEOPATH'S GUIDE TO KEEPING OUT OF TROUBLE

A toolkit to help meet professional obligations
and avoid pitfalls in practice

Paul Lambden

Radcliffe Publishing
Oxford • Seattle

Radcliffe Publishing Ltd
18 Marcham Road
Abingdon
Oxon OX14 1AA
United Kingdom

www.radcliffe-oxford.com
Electronic catalogue and worldwide online ordering facility.

British Library Cataloguing in Publication Data

A catalogue record for this book is available from the British Library.

ISBN 1 85775 737 8

Typeset by Anne Joshua & Associates, Oxford
Printed and bound by TJ International Ltd, Padstow, Cornwall

CONTENTS

PREFACE

Clinical practice has undergone a huge change over the last 30 years. It all used to be so simple. The patient would come to the surgery and explain to the osteopath the nature of the problem. The osteopath would examine the patient and notify the patient of what he (or occasionally she) had found. Treatment would then be prescribed and the necessary work undertaken. Patients would be unquestioning and grateful for whatever therapy they received. If the osteopath had an urge to explain in some detail to the patient what approach was anticipated, the patient would more than likely have waved the explanation away with a cheery, 'whatever you think, doc'. The osteopath would jot down a few, probably illegible, notes.

How different it all is now. We work in a litigious environment where adverse outcomes are viewed seriously. Osteopaths must be sure that they take careful histories, examine according to best practice, explain in sufficient detail the problem to be able to obtain valid consent, treat the patient with care and write notes that are sufficiently full and legible to ensure that the osteopath has a defence if a patient tries to take him (or her) to court.

It is probable that the treatment of today is of a much higher quality than a generation ago, but we have all paid a price to get it. Clinical work is now generally a much more stressful activity than it was in the past. The advent of risk management has hopefully started to reduce the risk of anything going wrong during clinical work and this book is an attempt to identify some of those areas where relatively simple changes may keep you safe, and where a bit of knowledge of the law and some simple ethical principles may support you in difficult times.

I have tried to keep the text relatively light and to avoid excessive detail. I have written it from the perspective of a medico-legal adviser. The availability of a trained medico-legal adviser at the other end of a telephone when a problem arises is often invaluable. The adviser can act as friend, adviser, supporter, confidant(e) and ally and his or her experience can often get an osteopath out of trouble quickly and efficiently.

Howden Insurance Services, for which I work, has recognised the huge value of effective medico-legal advice in times of trouble. Howden provides a high-quality insurance policy and it is a privilege to work with an organisation committed to excellence.

If you have any questions or nice comments about this book, please e-mail me at paullambden@compuserve.com – if you have any rude comments please keep them to yourself, because I am easily wounded.

Enjoy the book.

Paul Lambden
March 2005

ABOUT THE AUTHOR

Dr Paul Lambden BSc MB BS BDS FDSRCSEng MRCS(Eng) LRCP(Lond) DRCOG MHSM graduated in Medicine, Dentistry and Science at Guy's Hospital, London. After working initially in Oral Surgery and obtaining his Fellowship of the Royal College of Surgeons of England, he entered general medical and general dental practice, continuing the two for over 15 years. He was also a clinical tutor at St Bartholomew's Hospital, London.

In 1992 he left general practice to become the Chief Executive of East Hertfordshire NHS Trust, a whole district trust providing services for 300 000 people with a budget of over £65 million. He was also appointed a specialist adviser to the all-party Parliamentary Health Select Committee, which post he fulfilled for three years. In the late 1990s he became the Medical and Dental Principal of The St Paul International Insurance Company when it launched its professional indemnity (medical defence) programme for doctors and dentists. More recently he has worked as managing director of MIA General Insurance and is currently working at Howden Medical Insurance Services. He has recently been appointed Lecturer in Law and Ethics at the Kigezi International School of Medicine at Cambridge.

Paul is a regular writer on healthcare, management and medical defence topics. He has made a number of programmes for medical television channels and has been the author or co-author of half a dozen textbooks, including such subjects as the internet, law and ethics, the Human Rights Act and risk management in medicine and dentistry, and contributor to several more. He is a *Star Trek* fan.

DEDICATION

To Roy Lilley, my colleague and friend, with whom it has been my pleasure and privilege to write a number of books over recent years. He has taught me more about writing and communication than anyone else.

ACKNOWLEDGEMENTS

I am most grateful to Vincent Cullen, Head of Development at the General Osteopathic Council, to Charles Hunt, Vice Principal at the British School of Osteopathy, and to Paula Fletcher, Principal at the European School of Osteopathy, for their invaluable contributions, their peer review and proofreading skills. The views expressed in the book are not necessarily theirs and they have given generously of their advice in a personal capacity only. Also my thanks to Elizabeth Blanchfield of Howden Insurance for her considerable assistance with the Health and Safety sections, and to Asgar Hassanali, also of Howden Insurance, for his advice on some of the sections.

Insurance to protect and support osteopaths in circumstances where they are accused of negligence, poor practice or inappropriate conduct is referred to as **'professional indemnity'** throughout the book. The old term, 'medical malpractice', is now in my view considered obsolete, if only because of the insulting implication that the practitioner must have done something wrong. It should be consigned to history.

INTRODUCTION

It is likely that you will have neither the time nor the inclination to read any book from cover to cover, particularly one that includes risk, law and ethics. Frankly a bigger turn-off is hard to imagine.

So, to pander to those who have low boredom thresholds, short attention spans or lots of other interests, this book is divided into short, distinct sections, each of which can be read in isolation. There is no obligation to read more than a few pages at a time. Handy if you want to look at it between patients, in the bath, on the loo or during the adverts on television.

Some of it will be of no interest to you. Skip past those bits. Pick out those parts that look as though they may actually be useful. Make sure that the kettle is on and that you have a nice biscuit to go with the tea or coffee that you make regularly. Indeed, now seems a good time to make a cup of coffee and just have a flick through the book.

Welcome back! You will have noticed that law, ethics and risk management do not appear as separate sections. Frankly this is because they are in some parts too boring and the only way to really make them come alive is to apply each to the others to give an overall picture of how they work. You may also have spotted that the theories of ethics and the details of the law are also missing. They are omitted on the 'you don't need to understand an engine to drive a car' principle. The text is peppered with boxes of various sorts that are designed not only to break up the text, but to give you pause for thought.

Think boxes are there to get you thinking outside the box. Some of them are there to make you think, some, I hope, are provocative and some are there for a bit of fun.

Hazard warnings indicate tricky issues or traps that you should avoid for your own safety.

Tips are short cuts and quick fixes that will hopefully get you to an answer more quickly.

Exercises are issues for you to address and to use for brainstorming, for discussion with colleagues, or just to help you get your ideas straight.

Make a note is a comment designed to remind you of particular things that need to be done.

It is often the case that there is no straightforward answer to a simple question. It is my hope that this book will answer those questions that can be answered and perhaps point you in the right direction on those that are more tricky.

Before using this book you had better understand what it is that the book covers. So let's define what the components actually are.

The term 'Risk management' is made up of two words:

- *Risk* (n. & v.) – n. A chance or possibility of danger. Loss, injury or other adverse consequence.
- *Management* – n. The professional administration of business concerns.
- *Risk management* – Incomprehensible guru-speak and a task that is some-one else's job.

This has certainly been the traditional view, but the real definition is as follows:

- *Risk management* is a quality control related discipline comprising activities designed to minimise the adverse effects of loss upon a healthcare professional's physical, professional and financial assets by identifying any potential loss and reducing or preventing it.

It is helpful to define ethics and law as well.

- *Ethics* is the science of the morals of human conduct and provides the principles that rule the behaviour of society.
- *Law* is the enactment of custom or statute which is recognised as permitting or prohibiting certain actions and which is enforced by the imposition of penalties.

The strand that links ethics, law and risk is that registered osteopaths provide a standard expected by society, identified by ethics, upheld by law and with breaches minimised by risk management.

So Dear Reader, read on. Throw away any bits you don't want. Roll them up into a small ball and throw them at a picture of your bête noire, probably a tiresome patient or the local Inland Revenue inspector.

And *good luck*.

RISK MANAGEMENT

There is no doubt that claims are increasing. They are doing so for a variety of reasons:

- The population is more litigious and less tolerant of a medical outcome that is less than ideal.
- It has become much more fashionable to complain.
- The Government encourages complaints about healthcare.
- The media repeatedly provide programmes about poor healthcare, and advertisements for the 'where there's blame, there's a claim' culture stimulate dissatisfaction.
- The advent of no-win, no-fee arrangements.

Osteopaths do not have to succumb to the view that a claim is inevitable. By applying some simple risk management principles the likelihood of a complaint or a claim can be markedly reduced.

Risk management is a quality control related discipline comprising activities designed to minimise the adverse effects of loss upon a healthcare professional's physical, professional and financial assets by identifying any potential loss and reducing or preventing it.

There are four simple Principles of Risk Management:

☺ As a starter, have a look at your practice and see what risks you are exposed to – the dodgy electric plug, the dangling wire, the curly edge of a carpet. It takes 10 minutes and may save a fortune!

1 Identify the risk: what can go wrong?
2 Analyse the risk: how likely is it to go wrong and how serious an impact might it have?
3 Control the risk: what can I do to reduce or eliminate it or transfer it to someone else?
4 Cost the risk: what is the cost of getting it right versus the cost of getting it wrong?

Where studies have been undertaken it is clear that spending some time identifying and reducing risk pays dividends in terms of costs and time later on.

Furthermore, a claim from a damaged patient has not only financial consequences but often severe personal and emotional consequences as well.

Increased exposure to risk may occur for a variety of reasons:

- not being up to date with the latest best practice or technology
- managing badly a situation where a complication develops with a patient's care
- a failure of continuity of care
- a breakdown in communication
- failure to act to maintain the practice's assets
- failure to manage finance properly
- actions that lead to damage to reputation
- actions that lead to damage to relationships with family, colleagues or staff.

> ☑ It is everyone's job to be aware of risk management. Encourage it, support it, reward it and be pleased if all around you notice hazards that may be eliminated.

> ☑ Try the Post-It Note Challenge. Give some post-it notes to everyone in the practice, ask them to go round the building making a note and sticking a post-it note on everything that appears hazardous. You might be surprised by the result!

It is everyone's job to reduce or eliminate the risks associated with practice. Only by doing so will claims be kept under control and huge rises in insurance premiums be minimised. In some occupations bad claims histories already cause difficulty for the affected professionals in obtaining indemnity. And without insurance you cannot work.

> ☑ Remember that risk management is not just your job. It is the job of everyone involved in the practice.

In succeeding sections we shall look at areas where osteopaths are vulnerable to complaints and claims and suggest ways in which the risks can be reduced or removed.

THE DUTIES OF AN OSTEOPATH

The mainstream orthodox medical professions – including medicine, dentistry, osteopathy and chiropractic – have regulatory bodies and clear-cut codes of practice and standards. The codes for these four principal professions are remarkably similar and confer professional burdens on practitioners that are equally onerous. The operation of the General Osteopathic Council (GOsC) fulfils a number of functions:

- It protects patients by promoting excellence in osteopathic care.
- It regulates, develops and promotes the profession by:
  - maintaining a register of those osteopaths who are appropriately qualified and can demonstrate safe practice of the profession
  - defining standards of education, training and clinical practice
  - dealing promptly with osteopaths whose competence or fitness to practise is called into question
  - developing the profession and the practice of osteopathy.

The General Osteopathic Council produces *Pursuing Excellence*, a document which provides a code of practice for osteopaths. It outlines the principles under which every osteopath must operate. The code embraces the following statements:

- You must put patients first.
- You must foster and maintain trust between you and your patients.
- You must listen to patients and respect their views.
- You must give patients the information they need and be sure they understand you.
- You must respect and protect confidential information.
- You must respect patients' autonomy and allow them choice.

- You must maintain and develop your professional knowledge and skills.
- You must practise within your professional competence.
- You must never abuse your professional position.
- You must respect the skills of other healthcare professionals and work in co-operation with them.
- You must respond promptly and constructively to criticism and complaints.
- You must act quickly if you believe a colleague's conduct, health or professional performance, or your own, may pose a threat to patients.

After all this a cup of coffee is in order!

Complying with this code is demanding. It requires actions and behaviour of the highest standards. Yet the profession would not be able to act without such standards. Patients must trust osteopaths. They must feel sure that they understand what will happen to them and that information they provide will be kept secure. As skills evolve, all professionals must keep up to date and compliments and complaints should both receive prompt responses.

Finally, and perhaps most harshly, the osteopath must be prepared to notify GOsC if he or she becomes aware of a practitioner who may damage patients or whose behaviour brings the profession into disrepute. Failure to meet this latter standard may have serious consequences for an osteopath. If a patient suffers harm as a result of a practitioner's incompetence or ill-health, and the deficiency is known to another osteopath, and that knowledge subsequently comes to light, the osteopath may find himself brought before GOsC to explain and justify why he or she did not make the report.

> ☺ Which of the following incidents or circumstances should you notify to the insurer?
> - A patient who develops numbness in her arm after a cervical manipulation.
> - Someone who feels that you have breached confidentiality to his wife.
> - Someone who claims that you have undertaken treatment for which she did not consent.
> - A patient who had symptoms suggestive of a spinal tumour but whom you forgot to refer to a specialist for two weeks.
>
> ANSWER: All of them, of course. If anything at all happens, let the insurance company know.

The punishment for failure to report could be as severe as that for the osteopath whose performance was compromised.

It is the code of practice that holds the profession in good stead with society and which elevates the practitioners above those complementary and peripheral healthcare professions where questions of quality and standard remain unresolved because no such codes exist.

Will my premiums rise if I report several 'incidents'?

There is a common misconception that insurers are ready to pounce and increase premiums in such circumstances. However, practitioners whose bills are likely to rise are those whose claims are the result of repeated negligence or incompetence. Remember, too, that early advice reduces your risk of a claim developing. It is, in any case, a duty with any insurance policy to report events when they arise.

PROFESSIONAL INDEMNITY REQUIREMENTS

Osteopaths have seen some dramatic changes in their indemnity arrangements in recent years. Prices have risen rapidly as the number of claims has increased. In 2003 the Medical Protection Society, a medical defence organisation providing cover on a discretionary basis, briefly entered the market but withdrew because it could not comply with the requirements of the Osteopaths Act, which requires osteopaths to be insured. Last year, 2004, saw a large rise in premiums by one of the indemnity providers. It is tempting to ask why the market is so volatile and how claims are managed.

Indemnity may be provided within the insurance industry either on a *claims-made* or an *occurrence* basis. With a claims-made arrangement, the policy responds to a *claim*. The term 'claim' is really a poor term because it implies that the insurer is only interested in situations where an osteopath receives a solicitor's letter alleging professional misconduct or where the General Osteopathic Council notifies the osteopath of a complaint.

The insurer's interest is in fact much wider. It is a requirement to notify the company, not only about events such as those above but also about patient complaints made verbally or in writing to the osteopath, about enquiries from patients or legal firms for copies or sight of the osteopathic records (using the Data Protection Act 1998) and of any incident or circumstance that might later give rise to any sort of claim.

By contrast an occurrence-based policy provides indemnity depending on when the 'incident' occurred. The event in question may have taken place months or years earlier but as long as the insurance was in place at the time of the incident the osteopath can seek cover under the policy. An occurrence insurer needs to be notified of all the same events and incidents.

A number of questions arise from these arrangements.

IS A CLAIMS-MADE OR AN OCCURRENCE POLICY BETTER?

In reality both types of policy meet the requirements of the policyholders to respond to claims provided the appropriate arrangements are in place. However, there is a key difference.

A *claims-made* policy responds to a 'claim'. At the end of any policy year the insurer will have received notification of a number of claims as a result of allegations against osteopaths. All the claims will either have been resolved (successfully defended or settled) or reserved (an estimate made of the likely final costs involved in handling the claim). The insurer will therefore have a good understanding of the total financial liability to which it will be exposed and can allocate funds to meet the claims accordingly. It is also able to ensure the appropriate setting of premium for the following year.

Occurrence-based indemnity provides cover based on the date when the 'incident', rather than the claim, actually occurred. The claim associated with any incident may arise weeks, months or years later. It is possible that a claim could arise 10 years or more after the event and some claims arise 'out of the blue' with no prior warning that an 'incident' has occurred. This might make reserve forecasting (putting aside sufficient money to meet claims that may arise in future) difficult for an insurer because, at the end of a policy year, it will not have a clear idea whether it will receive further claims in the future and, if so, what their value will be.

WHAT IS 'RUN OFF'?

Run off is cover provided by an insurer to meet claims that may arise in the future after the active policy has been terminated. If a policyholder ceases to have insurance, there could be a risk that a claim could be made for which he or she did not have cover unless appropriate arrangements had been made. There has on occasion been a problem with osteopaths leaving a claims-made insurer. In that situation some osteopaths have been asked to pay an additional charge for future cover. In fact this is *not necessary* for osteopaths moving to another claims-made insurer with retrospective cover and may be another benefit of the claims-made policy. Because a claims-made policy looks at when the *claim* is made, the incident may have occurred before the osteopath was insured. Provided the osteopath was unaware of any potential claim at the time he or she took the insurance, the policy will respond to any appropriate claim, subject to the terms of the policy, as long as it occurs during the period of insurance. An occurrence policy only operates provided it was in force when the incident occurred.

How is a 'claim' managed?

The insurer will provide assistance and support when any incidents or circumstances are notified. For those osteopaths insured through Howden, the medico-legal team will work with the claims team of the insurance company that underwrites the cover to ensure that the osteopath receives all necessary advice to react quickly. Where it will be necessary to manage a claim and seek legal advice, all arrangements will be made by the insurance company with medico-legal input and the osteopath will be informed and involved at all stages.

Why was The Medical Protection Society not able to provide indemnity for osteopaths?

The Medical Protection Society was unable to provide indemnity because it is a mutual society providing discretionary cover and the Osteopath's Act 1993 requires the General Council 'to secure that they are properly insured against liabilities to, or in relation to, their patients'. Because the indemnity provided by the MPS is discretionary there is no contractual obligation to meet a claim but only a promise that cover will be considered. Chiropractors must also have insurance rather than discretionary cover by law although doctors and dentists are permitted to have discretionary indemnity in the United Kingdom.

Any high-quality insurer will have as its aim to provide high-quality, rapid assistance to the policyholders. Insurers understand how distressing a claim may be and how important it is to be able to speak to another healthcare professional whenever it is necessary. If you have any concerns or problems associated with your professional activities, be sure your cover is provided by an insurer offering *medico*-legal support.

HANDLING COMPLAINTS

Complaints are on the increase across the whole spectrum of healthcare. Most complaints received by osteopaths are dealt with within the practice. Only a relatively small number go on to become a claim or are lodged with the General Osteopathic Council. Receipt of a complaint is an important event. It must be handled effectively. Some authorities say that complaints are good and should be treated as a learning exercise. Others think they are a nuisance to be cleared as quickly as possible. Whatever the viewpoint, a dissatisfied complainant can cause a lot of trouble for an osteopath.

Ten top tips for complaint handling
1 Keep the insurer informed
2 Do not ignore complaints
3 Act quickly
4 Speak to the patient
5 Do not write aggressive responses
6 Do not miss out difficult bits
7 A conciliator may help
8 Do not get cross
9 It may be OK to return fees
10 It may be OK to say sorry

Best practice suggests that the following principles should always be adopted:

1 *Keep your insurer informed:* At those insurers with medico-legal advisers, they are used to dealing with complaints. It is often the case that the person to whom the complaint has been directed is the last person to respond in a calm and rational manner. You should telephone the advice line

✎ Insurers are set up to help with complaints. Let them know straight away if you get one. They understand that even the best osteopath can get a complaint and it is not seen as an automatic black mark. However, hiding a complaint may be regarded as original sin.

to find out the best course of action. You should receive advice on the reply and a review of your draft response letter to make sure that it uses appropriate wording. If you don't, change your insurer!

2 *Do not ignore complaints:* A complaint does not go away. Do not put it in a drawer and hope that you will not hear any more. You will, and next time it will be more aggressive and difficult to deal with.

3 *Act quickly:* The evidence is that a speedy response is much more likely to resolve a problem than a slow one peppered with delays.

4 *Speak to the patient:* Although this advice is not ideal in every case, it is held that in most cases speaking to a dissatisfied patient can contribute to resolving the problem. Talking to people – communicating – is what all healthcare professionals do and you should be very good at it. It is also important not to forget that complainants may have some justification for complaint and you never know, you might even learn something.

5 *Do not write aggressive responses:* Telling a patient what you think of them in a complaint response may make you feel better, but it will be short-lived. The patient is very likely to write again, this time more aggressively and will also be more prepared to complain to others, such as GOsC.

If you are going to respond aggressively you must be sure that

🖎 Healthcare professionals are expert at talking to patients, especially when the patients are cross or upset. Unless there is a good reason *not* to talk to someone, it is well worth the effort. If you do, do so in a relaxed atmosphere, offer them a cup of tea, have someone present (a receptionist or practice manager) taking notes (and who will give a copy of the notes to both you and the patient afterwards) and talk through the problem.

Talk through the strategy with the insurer beforehand.

Light relief

Handling complaints is an art. Patient complaints are often colourful and the following caused consternation when they were received in letters:

- 'The osteopath's suggestion that the diagnosis would only be made at post-mortem was entirely unacceptable.'
- 'When I tried to make an appointment I discovered you were on holiday. The receptionist refused to give me your holiday address.'
- 'To be told that people as old and fat as me should not go to the gym was abrupt to the point of offence.'

you are absolutely right and that you have no regard for any con-sequences. Such consequences could be regulatory body interest, bad publicity and damage to reputation. Remember also for whom the letter is written. *Although it may be addressed to an individual who has complained, the likelihood is that it will be shown to others*: friends, relatives, Citizens Advice Bureau, etc. The complainant may even agree (at least privately) with what you have said but it may not sound so good to others who were less personally involved.

6 *Do not miss out difficult bits:* It is often the case that a complaint letter raises a number of issues. Even if one or more of the matters is embarrassing or difficult it is unwise to leave it out in the hope that detailed answers to more minor complaints will distract the patient from the key issue. It will not. You will simply receive a further letter specifically directed to the difficult complaint, which will then be more awkward to answer effectively.

> **Oh dear**
>
> Sadly, replies in draft responses are often not useable:
> - 'I am well-known for my obtuse manner.'
> - 'I am naturally disappointed that my manipulation of your lumbar spine was ineffective but pleased that your appendicectomy was successful.'
> - 'If I ever see you again it will be much too soon!'

7 *A conciliator:* Sometimes personality conflicts prevent an osteopath negotiating a resolution with a patient. In such circumstances a colleague or other individual may be able to act as a conciliator to bring about a conclusion to the complaint. If you are struggling with a complaint, discuss the possibilities with your insurance company medico-legal advisers.

8 *Don't get cross:* This is really the ultimate sign of failure. If you lose your temper everything will break down and the complainant may well pass the issue on to someone else. The someone else may be GOsC or a lawyer.

9 *It may be OK to return fees:* There is often much concern about whether it is appropriate to return fees. In many cases complainants ask for return of fees if a treatment(s) has not worked. Sometimes outcomes are such that osteopaths themselves want to return fees, either because they recognise things have not achieved desired results or simply to get rid of the patient. If a return of fees is an issue:
- Discuss it with your insurance company medico-legal adviser.
- It is reasonable to return fees in circumstances where you believe that to do so may bring about a resolution to a problem. In such

circumstances it should be done as a *gesture of goodwill* and *without admission of liability*.

10 *It may be OK to say sorry:* Healthcare practitioners are often unsure whether to say sorry. It all depends on the circumstances. It is reasonable to apologise for those circumstances for which you would apologise in any non-clinical situation, e.g. 'I am sorry that you had to go to the hospital', or 'I'm sorry that you had the pain'. Such comments are simply those that a reasonable person would make.

What you should not do is to apologise for your treatment. '*I am sorry that I got the diagnosis wrong*' or '*I am sorry I made a mess of your treatment*' could be disastrous comments, especially when feeling remorse about an adverse outcome. In any case it often occurs that treatments that seem, on the face of things, to have been inappropriate in the light of the outcome may be regarded as reasonable when reviewed by other osteopaths. You must remember that no one can do everything right all the time and, in any case, you are not clairvoyant. What you must do is to use your professional skills to make a reasonable assessment of the patient and to provide the standard of care of an osteopath ordinarily skilled in the treatment being provided.

If you get a complaint tell your insurance company medico-legal adviser. Get help to manage the complaint and write the reply. If you can satisfy the patient and resolve the complaint you will have a less stressful practising life and a much lower risk of a claim. After all, you don't want to meet a lawyer, do you?

THE GENERAL OSTEOPATHIC COUNCIL

The General Osteopathic Council (GOsC) is the regulatory body for osteopaths. All osteopaths must be registered with GOsC to be able to practise, and for the privilege of registration they must pay an annual retention fee.

The osteopathic profession, like the other mainstream healthcare professions, enjoys self-regulation. In other words, the regulation of the profession is done by the profession rather than by an outside agency. The Government has recently created statutory bodies such as the Council for Healthcare Regulatory Excellence (CHRE) and the National Clinical Assessment Authority (NCAA), both of which have powers to intervene with the regulatory procedure but, currently, these regulatory procedures still substantially remain with the regulatory bodies such as GOsC. More of this later!

For most osteopaths GOsC is regarded as an organisation that takes a subscription annually and causes them problems if a patient complains about them. From an insurance point of view, it is important not to incur the interest of GOsC if at all possible because hearings are traumatic for the osteopath and expensive for the insurer (with consequent implications for future premiums). The role of the Council should be understood.

The Council regulates and monitors osteopaths' fitness to practise. It is an integral part of the Council's duties to regulate the profession and protect the public and the profession's reputation. Under Section 20 of the Osteopaths Act 1993, GOsC has legal powers to consider cases where it is alleged that an osteopath has been guilty of professional misconduct or incompetence, convicted of a criminal offence or impaired by health problems. Such allegations are reviewed through a series of committees: the *Investigating Committee*, the *Professional Conduct Committee* and the *Health Committee*.

Any concern about fitness to practise can be raised with GOsC. Usually complaints come from the public, but the police have an obligation to report to GOsC any osteopath convicted of a criminal offence. There is also an increasing duty on other healthcare professionals to notify GOsC of any osteopath whose practice gives cause for concern. Furthermore, checks will be made on the criminal records of all osteopaths on the Osteopath Register.

If a complaint is made to the Council it is first reviewed by a *screener*. The screener will decide whether the complaint falls within the GOsC's remit. If it does not do so, the complainant will be informed accordingly. If it is within GOsC's responsibility, it will be referred to the *Investigating Committee* for further consideration together with a report from the screener. A copy of the complaint will be sent to the osteopath. A response to the allegation may be made within 28 days. *If an osteopath receives a letter from GOsC notifying him or her about a complaint and asking for observations, it is absolutely essential that insurance advisers are notified immediately.* The osteopath's response may be sent to the complainant for further comments and, in the event that more information is provided by the complainant, the osteopath has a further opportunity to make additional observations. The Investigating Committee may also seek any other information that it considers necessary, for example GP or hospital notes.

Once the Investigating Committee decides that it has collected all the information that it requires from the complainant and the osteopath, it decides what further action it should take. To decide to take action it must conclude that there is sufficient evidence of:

- unacceptable professional conduct
- professional incompetence
- a relevant criminal offence
- health issues.

It may decide that there is *no case to answer*, in which circumstance the case is closed and the osteopath notified. It is, however, important to note that GOsC may keep the complaint on file and can reactivate it if a further case of a similar nature is reported within a set time.

If the Investigating Committee decides that there *is a case to answer* it formulates the allegations and may then refer the osteopath to the *Professional Conduct Committee* or, if the osteopath is believed to be unwell and the ability to practise is seriously impaired because of mental or physical health, to the *Health Committee*.

If the Investigating Committee decides that the allegations are of such seriousness that the osteopath may represent a danger to the public, it has the power to order the Registrar to suspend the osteopath's registration. The osteopath is notified by the Investigating Committee that an interim suspension hearing will be held to decide whether he or she may continue to practise. The osteopath may attend and can represent him or herself or be represented by a lawyer or medico-legal adviser. If the decision is made to suspend the osteopath, he or she can no longer practise whilst the investigations continue.

Most *Professional Conduct Committee* cases are considered within three to six months although delays may occur if there is a police investigation where the Council cannot proceed until it is concluded. Cases heard by the Professional Conduct Committee are often very intimidating for osteopaths. They are quasi-judicial and both sides are represented by lawyers. The evidence is presented for both sides and witnesses are examined. The osteopath's own evidence will be presented by questioning from the barrister acting for the osteopath and he or she will be cross-examined by the barrister acting for the Council. When the case is complete the Committee, which is comprised of a mixture of lay members and professional osteopath members, withdraws to consider its decision. The Committee can exonerate the osteopath or can establish that the case is well-founded, finding the osteopath guilty of either *unacceptable professional conduct* or *professional incompetence*. In such circumstances the Committee has a range of sanctions that can be applied. They are:

- Erasure from the register.
- Suspension from the register for a period of time.
- The application of Conditions on Practice. Such conditions might be, for example, that the osteopath should always have a chaperone or not provide treatment for anyone under the age of 16.
- The application of conditions on the osteopath. Such conditions might be, for example, a period of re-training or postgraduate refreshment in particular areas of skill. Sometimes the osteopath is ordered to have a mentor for a period.
- Admonishment.

Hearings of the Professional Conduct Committee are usually complete within one year, although they occasionally take longer in circumstances where, for example, additional evidence is made available.

The *Health Committee* is convened and considers cases where it is alleged that an osteopath's ability to practise is seriously impaired because of his physical or mental health. The Health Committee also consists of a mixture of lay and osteopath members. In some circumstances the committee can consider a case using only the paperwork submitted without the need to bring the osteopath before the committee, in circumstances where both parties are content that such an approach can be adopted. In those cases where a hearing is required it is done in private because of the personal confidential nature of the medical evidence that is involved.

After hearing the evidence the Health Committee members will decide whether it is their view that the osteopath's ability to practise is seriously impaired by his physical or mental health. If they decide affirmatively, then they may take one of the following actions:

- Suspend the osteopath's registration for a set period.
- Impose conditions on the osteopath's practice.

The Health Committee has no power to erase an osteopath from the register. In general the committee will review the osteopath at regular intervals to decide whether his or her health status has improved sufficiently to enable a return to normal practice.

Figure 1			
	2001	*2002*	*2003*
Unprofessional conduct	4	12	5
Incompetence	0	3	1
Criminal convictions	0	0	0
Health incapacity	0	1	0

In circumstances where a judgement is made against an osteopath, he or she has the right to appeal to the High Court or to seek a judicial review.

Fortunately, cases before the General Osteopathic Council are relatively rare. Only exceptionally is an osteopath suspended or erased from the register. The cases to answer between 2001 and 2003 are as illustrated in Figure 1.

AVOIDING THE GENERAL OSTEOPATHIC COUNCIL

A review of the cases that appear before the Professional Conduct Committee repeatedly suggests that simple procedures or actions could have avoided any difficulties. The five things of which osteopaths should be most aware are as follows:

1 *Consent:* Be certain that you have adequately explained your treatment plan to the patient and that the patient has given a valid consent for you

to provide that treatment. The more intrusive the treatment proposed, the more detailed must be the explanation.

☢   Patients can be dangerous. Don't let them expose you to risk. Be careful.

2 *Respect privacy and dignity:* Ensure that patients can undress and dress in private areas.

3 *Availability of a chaperone:* Ensure that you have a chaperone available if required and that every patient can have access to a chaperone if they wish to have one. If you do not have suitable staff or colleagues available, you should consider inviting the patient to return at another time, bringing with them their own friend or relative to act as a chaperone.

4 *Ensure your notes are adequate:* Remember that they are often your only defence in cases where an allegation is made years after the incident.

5 *Do not have personal intimate relationships with your patients:* If you detect any improper advances on the part of patients you should clearly reject them and decline to see the patient again. If you feel that there is any risk that a professional relationship might at some stage in the future become more personal, you should terminate the professional relationship imme-diately and make clear that you have done so.

As with all incidents and cir-cumstances, if you receive any notification from GOsC of any complaint from any source, you should immediately notify your insurance company medico-legal adviser, who will provide assistance in managing the matter.

Thought for the day

Spare a thought for GOsC. These days they find themselves in something of a dilemma. If they are too tough on osteo-paths, they end up being criticised by the profession, but if they are too leni-ent, the Council for Healthcare Regula-tory Excellence (CHRE) has the power to review the case and, if it feels that GOsC has not issued a suitable punish-ment, take it to the High Court.

THE COUNCIL FOR HEALTHCARE REGULATORY EXCELLENCE (CHRE)

The CHRE, established by the Government, is seen by many as a threat to the self-regulation of the nine statutory healthcare regulators in the United Kingdom. It was established in April 2003 and its remit is:

- to promote the interests of the public and patients in relation to regulation of the healthcare professions
- to promote best practice in the regulation of the healthcare professions
- to develop principles for good professionally-led regulation
- to promote co-operation between regulatory bodies and other organisations.

The CHRE is an overarching, independent body that overseas the regulatory work of the nine regulating bodies: the General Medical Council, General Dental Council, General Osteopathic Council, General Chiropractic Council, General Optical Council, The Health Professions Council, The Nursing and Midwifery Council, The Royal Pharmaceutical Society of Great Britain and the Pharmaceutical Society of Northern Ireland. It is accountable to Parliament in Westminster and independent of the UK Departments of Health.

The significance for practitioners is that it has the power to appeal decisions of the regulatory bodies. If a decision by GOsC finding a practitioner not guilty of serious professional misconduct is a 'relevant decision' it can be referred to court by CHRE under Section 29(4) of the National Health Service Reform and Health Care Professions Act 2002. This effectively means that the CHRE can challenge 'not guilty' findings as well as unduly lenient sanctions.

Many authorities regard this power as wholly unacceptable because a practitioner so treated will in effect be exposed to a double jeopardy effect, having to defend him or herself in a regulatory body hearing, only to be subject to the possibility of referral and review of the whole case again by the High Court if found to be innocent or only guilty of a more minor offence. I hope that the CHRE does not represent a Government-sponsored system for more draconian judgements for osteopaths and other healthcare professionals or the beginning of the end for self-regulation.

COMPETENCE AND CONTINUING PROFESSIONAL DEVELOPMENT

Competence is a central concept in all healthcare professions. If an osteopath acts in a way that suggests or demonstrates that he or she lacks the competence to satisfactorily undertake his or her job, then the likelihood is that he or she will end up before a GOsC hearing and may be required to undergo retraining or, in extreme cases, may be erased from the register. In modern parlance the term 'capability' is being increasingly used in preference to competence.

Standard 2000 (S2K) provides a framework for review and is arranged within 16 areas of capability. They integrate the areas of professional knowledge, personal capabilities and occupational capabilities. The areas of capability are as follows:

1 knowledge to provide safe and competent practice of osteopathy
2 concepts and principles of osteopathy
3 therapeutic and professional relationships
4 personal and individual skills
5 communication skills
6 information and data handling skills
7 intra- and interprofessional collaboration and co-operation
8 professional identity and accountability, ethics and responsibilities
9 professional self-evaluation and development by means of reflective practice

10 identification and evaluation of the needs of the patient
11 acquisition and enhancement of the skills of osteopathic palpation
12 planning, justifying and monitoring osteopathic treatment interventions
13 conducting osteopathic treatment and patient management
14 evaluation of post-treatment progress and change

> ☢ Every healthcare profession is going through a tightening of continuing professional development. Think about it now before it becomes a burden. Training is in two parts: doing it and proving that you have done it. The second is sometimes more difficult than the first.

15 advice and support for the promotion and maintenance of healthy living
16 managing an efficient and effective environment for the provision of osteopathic healthcare.

This list looks daunting. It is hard to imagine how to maintain adequate skills and capability in all these areas without undergoing training for several weeks a year. But actually it isn't as traumatic as it looks. Every osteopath will know much of what is required and it is a matter of tailoring continuing professional development to ensure that any gaps in knowledge are plugged.

Consider those 16 areas of capability and tick off what you already know. You will be pleasantly surprised. Much of it is in the book and some of the areas covered have been ticked off for you.

General capability	Specific area	✓
Knowledge relevant to safe and competent practice of osteopathy	Anatomy, especially with respect to the neuro-muscular system	
	Sociology and psychology	
	Clinical reasoning and decision-making skills	
	General medical knowledge	
	Managing people	✓
Concepts and principles of osteopathy	General principles	
	Osteopathic techniques	
Therapeutic and professional relationships	Ethical issues associated with professional practice	✓
	Management of uncertainty	
	Managing the difficult patient	✓
	Ensuring confidentiality	✓
	Obtaining valid consent	✓
Personal and individual skills	Awareness of strengths and weaknesses	
	Problem-solving skills	
	Ability to self-direct learning	
	Awareness of self-protection	✓

General capability	Specific area	✓
Communication skills	Awareness of nature and variety of communication skills	✓
Information and data handling	Adequate IT skills	
	Basic word processing skills	
	Ability to use spreadsheets	
	Financial management	
	Audit and research	
Collaboration and co-operation	Critical appraisal	
	Understanding of the NHS	
	Awareness of complementary medicine	
	Understanding referral criteria	
	Understanding of multi-professional planning	
Identity, ethics and responsibilities	Understanding of self-regulation	
	Understanding safety and self-assessment of competence	✓
	Legal responsibilities	✓
	Ethical behaviour	✓
	Maintaining the reputation of the profession	✓
Self-evaluation and reflective practice	Compliance with CPD requirements	✓
	Recording self-monitoring	
	Participation in relevant structured courses and conferences	
	Involvement in group activities	
	Ability to generate self-audit	
	Ability to contribute to research	
Evaluation of the needs of the patient	Effective and efficient case history preparation	
	Analysis of patient complaints	
	Knowledge of clinical investigations	
	Ability to examine patients	
	Ability to formulate differential diagnosis	
	Consulting with the patient	
	Minority issues	
	Good record keeping	✓
	Good referral letters	
Enhancement of skills of osteopathic palpation	Therapeutic value of touch and palpation	
	Advanced knowledge of palpatory characteristics of tissues	
Planning, justifying and monitoring treatment interventions	Good history taking	✓
	Rational decision-making	
	To treat or not to treat	
	Treatment planning	
	Advising and informing patients	
	Therapeutic contracts	
Treatment and patient management	Selection of techniques	
	Theories, principles and practice of osteopathy	
Evaluation of progress and change	Reviewing responses to treatment	
	Assessing continuation plans	
	Adverse reaction recognition	

General capability	Specific area	✓
Promotion of healthy living	Appreciation of concepts Informed patient choices about healthy living Assisting patients with self-care activities	
Offering an efficient environment for providing osteopathic care	Legal requirements of modern practice Financial management Managing staff effectively Management and security of patient records	✓ ✓

Do you see what good value this book is? Reading it should be worth some CPD.

So what is required of the osteopath in respect of CPD? Indeed, what is CPD?

Continuing professional development is learning. It is as simple as that! The learning may take any form, structured or unstructured – lectures, seminars, clinical and theoretical training and anything else that helps in the acquisition of knowledge.

> **To find the GOsC document**
>
> Go to the Internet.
> Visit www.osteopathy.org.uk.
> This takes you to the home page.
> Click on *TRAINING AND CPD*.
> On the next page, click on *CPD*.
> On the next page click on: *Forming Knowledge – A guide to CPD for Osteopaths*.
> *It's all there, 43 pages of it!*

> ☢ You have to pay for all this training yourself. Watch out for free lectures and sponsored NHS events.

The General Osteopathic Council, like other regulatory bodies, has introduced a requirement for every osteopath, whether full-time, part-time or even non-practising (assuming they may want to do so again) of **30 hours** a year as a **minimum**. It started as standard for **all** osteopaths on 1 May 2004 so the first year ends on 30 April 2005. This is a trial period but, believe me, it will not be scrapped even if it is a disaster. What is more, if the scheme follows the same path as regulatory bodies, you can expect the conditions to be tightened.

GOsC has defined the CPD in two broad categories: personal learning and group learning (involving other osteopaths or other health professionals).

A minimum of **15 hours** must fall into each category. If asked, you must be able to justify your claims to have either studied on your own or attended lectures, etc. and you must make a declaration to the Council demonstrating the training you have undertaken. GOsC will monitor the compliance with the scheme although, interestingly, the scheme will not be used as an assessment of competence (though if you find yourself at GOsC accused of incompetence, being able to produce a folder showing a comprehensive variety of training over a period of time will be valuable support).

The choice of training is left to the osteopath but it must be relevant to the osteopathic practice (but excludes animal treatment). Don't think that you can have a raunchy weekend in a Swedish Massage Parlour and claim that it is all valuable study for use in your practice in Surbiton (I didn't pick Surbiton for any particular reason – it could be anywhere).

All this information is available in the GOsC document *Forming Knowledge*, which can be downloaded from the GOsC website.

Many healthcare professionals regard CPD as a chore. It is often not so much the doing it as having to write it down. After all, most osteopaths will do training every year. This is merely a formalisation of the process.

You must also maintain a CPD folder and you must keep the details of the training that you undertake for a minimum of **five years** after completion of the CPD year in question. The folder should look respectable, not some scruffy old folder that you previously used for something else with scribbled notes of study on bits of toilet paper shoved in it. The Portfolio should contain, for each element of study that you undertake, the following details:

- *Selection and planning:* The way in which you chose the course and how it fits in with your overall programme of study.
- *Justification of your selected activities:* You must explain how the course relates to your practice and what aspect of your work will be improved by spending the time doing the activity.
- *Evidence that you have completed the activities:* A certificate of attendance is good and most courses will provide such a document. Alternatively, signing in and enclosing details of the course. Ideally a photograph of you with the lecturer would be useful (only kidding!).
- *Evaluation of your learning:* An explanation of how the course (or whatever) relates to the activities you perform in your practice and how much better at them you will be after the training.

> ☢ The sting in the tail is that, if you fail to complete the annual training requirement and return the Annual Summary, you will not be able to practise legally as an osteopath. You will remain barred until you have met the conditions necessary to restore you to the register, subject to agreement from the registrar.

GOsC will in due course be issuing folders, using your subscriptions to fund them, but in the meantime the website document includes blank CPD forms that you can complete.

GOsC has the right to inspect your folder at any time (and they will do so in due course). If you receive such a request you should send a photocopy and **not** the original.

So good luck with your CPD. Actually it can be quite fun if you sign up for the right courses and you use the opportunity to kill two birds with one stone, i.e. meeting your obligations to retain your registration with GOsC and at the same time expanding your knowledge to improve your practice. If you have got any doubts or questions the *Forming Knowledge* document seems to answer everything you could think of, and a whole load of things you haven't thought of. So go for it and become a genius in osteopathy.

CLINICAL NEGLIGENCE

Clinical negligence is a term that is used to mean poor clinical practice of an unacceptable standard. It is in fact alleged wrongdoing in the area of expertise of a practitioner and may be challenged by the injured party in *civil* law. Allegations of negligence may be levied against an osteopath and, if made and refuted, can be judged in court.

> If you injure one of your patients and it is unquestionably your fault and you should have realised the risk when you did the treatment, a claim for negligence against you is almost bound to succeed and the insurer will want to settle it as quickly and cheaply as possible.

It is possible to raise proceedings against an osteopath under *tort*, which is interpersonal wrongdoing short of criminality. Action may also be taken under the *law of contract*, which deals with disputes arising from legally enforceable agreements.

For negligence to be demonstrated there is a requirement to be able to demonstrate that:

- the practitioner owed a duty of care to the person making the claim
- the duty of care was breached
- an injury was suffered
- the injury was the direct result of the breach of the duty of care (causation)
- the injury was foreseeable.

All these elements must be demonstrable if the claimant is to succeed in an allegation of negligence.

In addition, claims arising in private practice may be generated by alleged breach of contract as well as by negligence. A *contract* is an agreement creating obligations that are recognised and enforceable by law. For there to be a contract there must be:

- an offer
- an acceptance
- a consideration – the price (payment) for which the contract is bought.

Such an arrangement applies only to private practice. In NHS work no consideration passes between the NHS patient and the treating practitioner or hospital.

The duty of care is the professional obligation that an osteopath has to a patient and is enshrined in common law. Such a duty exists from the point at which a patient is accepted explicitly or implicitly. It is usually clear-cut although there are circumstances where the osteopath may find that his or her primary duty is to someone other than the patient. For example, an osteopath may be asked to write a report on a patient's condition for an insurance company or an employer. In such a circumstance the osteopath–patient relationship does not exist in conventional terms but the osteopath does still have a duty to comply with professional requirements and to avoid causing harm.

In negligence the practitioner has to demonstrate that what he or she did was appropriate and of an adequate standard. This is achieved by a judicial review of professional opinion to assess *the standard of care*. In other words, a practitioner cannot act in a certain way in the absolute knowledge that his or her actions could not subsequently be challenged and an allegation of negligence made.

In 1957 the *Bolam* case (*Bolam v Friern Hospital Management Committee*) established the essence of negligence by setting the standard for a breach of duty of care. The standard set was of the ordinarily skilled man exercising and professing to have that special skill. The man did not need to possess the highest expert skill in order to avoid being found guilty of negligence. For the law it was sufficient for him to exercise the ordinary skill of the ordinary competent man exercising that particular art.

The *Bolam* judgment followed a case two years earlier in Scotland when Lord President Clyde set out the definition for medical negligence in the case of *Hunter v Hanley*. He said: 'The true test for establishing negligence and diagnosis or treatment on the part of the doctor is whether he has been proved to be guilty of such failure as no doctor of ordinary skill would be guilty of if acting with ordinary care'. He later expanded this view by stating that liability could be established only with the demonstration of three factors: first, that there is a normal and usual practice; second, that the doctor had not adopted that practice; and third, that the course the doctor adopted is one that no professional man of ordinary skill would have taken.

Both in Scotland and England these judgments related to a negligence allegation involving a medical practitioner but the judgments have been rolled out across the whole spectrum of healthcare.

The clear message that emanates from these two cases is that acting reasonably to the standard of your peers gives a defence against an allegation of negligence.

Part of the success in a case of alleged negligence (in those cases that reach court) is that the experts impress the judge as being honest and reasonable. This factor was very important in a further case that has influenced the situation in respect of negligence: the *Bolitho* case (*Bolitho and others v City and Hackney Health Authority 1997*). This was a complicated case that went to the Court of Appeal and ultimately to the House of Lords and led to consideration of the issues surrounding the situation where experts acting for both sides both offered compelling arguments. The judge normally relies on the clinical evidence in order to make a judgment and, in such circumstances, he had to decide whether the experts acting for the claimant or the defendant submitted the more logical and sustainable arguments. In fact, in this case, the judges ultimately found for the defendant but the case laid down important criteria. It reinforced the paramount status of the *Bolam* case and *Hunter v Hanley*. It also made clear that experts must be of the highest calibre and be able to carefully consider the issues and articulate their views on a convincing basis.

In essence, *Bolitho*, whilst upholding the test of reasonableness, reminded the professions that, in circumstances where there is expert opinion on both sides, the judge must decide which body of opinion is more reasonable and convincing.

The **standard of proof** required in a civil case is that a particular event was more likely than not to have happened, i.e. the balance of probabilities as opposed to the criminal standard, which is beyond reasonable doubt.

Causation is a term used to describe whether an incident (whether through act or omission) if alleged to be negligent actually caused or materially contributed to a loss or injury. If an osteopath provides treatment and there is an adverse outcome, but it can be shown that the outcome would have been the same irrespective of whether the treatment had been provided, then the osteopath cannot be held to be negligent.

Many observers view the negligence situation as biased in favour of the healthcare practitioners, based on the *Bolam* and *Hunter v Hanley* judgments. In other words, they see as difficult the fact that the claimant (pursuer in Scotland) has to prove that the practitioner (defendant in England and Wales or defender in Scotland) breached the duty of care, specifically caused or contributed to the loss or injury in circumstances that were reasonably foreseeable and needs only to act to a reasonable standard of an ordinarily skilled practitioner rather than someone practising to the best standard possible. Many practitioners, particularly those who have been accused of negligence, may well say that things are difficult enough as they are.

Compensation for an injury in a civil claim can only be by the payment of money. Successful claimants are usually awarded **general** and **special** damages. Such settlements may be 'once-and-for-all' payments although they may be staged over a period of time, up to and including life. The potential payments are not entirely without conditions.

A claimant has a duty to mitigate the loss. In other words, if a claimant suffers an injury at the hands of an osteopath and appropriate corrective treatment may reduce or resolve the consequences or the suffering, then the treatment should not be delayed until the outcome of the trial is known or settlement reached before receiving the treatment in question. If a claimant refuses treatment that could have lessened the duration or consequences of the injury, then the claimant must demonstrate that his refusal to accept the treatment was reasonable.

General damages are awarded for the pain and suffering associated with the injury suffered. **Special damages** are awarded as a specific payment especially for the claimant's particular injury and the consequences that are the result of the injury. The damages may be calculated on a range of factors. Much of the claim will be associated with the costs associated with any immediate corrective treatment and any costs associated with further treatment that would be required in the future. However, other costs that can be added are such things as radiology, drug costs, travel costs and expert opinion paid for by the claimant, and even such things as special footwear or appliances. In a circumstance, for example, where an osteopath has injured a patient and the treatment of the injury required some sort of individually prepared supportive appliance, the appliance would be expected to wear out and the special damages would include a calculation based on the replacement cycle of the appliance, the person's life expectancy and the expected future cost of the device. A calculation is performed that should arrive at a lump sum which, when invested, would be expected to provide for the treatment costs over the claimant's lifetime. Claimants are entitled to the costs of *private* corrective treatment even though the same treatment might be available under the National Health Service. In successful cases claimants are also entitled to receive interest on damages awarded, calculated from the date of the clinical incident giving rise to the claim.

Compensation recovery may be influenced by the nature of the injury sustained. If the claimant has received state benefits as a result of the alleged injury, then these payments will be deducted from the eventual compensation by the **Compensation Recovery Unit** if the case is successful. In the case of a serious injury, in circumstances where the claimant is paid considerable compensation in excess of that allowed for capital holdings with certain means-tested benefits, he or she may not be able to receive those state benefits until their means dwindle. It is possible to circumvent this problem by placing the compensation in a special needs trust fund with the claimant as the only beneficiary.

Time for a lie down in a dark room, or perhaps a cuppa?

THE PROCESS OF THE LAW

The litigation process underwent a huge change following a review of the previous procedure by Lord Woolf, who was appointed to do so by the Lord Chancellor in 1994. The new **Civil Procedure Rules** came into effect in 1998. Their purposes were:

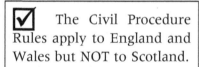

☑   The Civil Procedure Rules apply to England and Wales but NOT to Scotland.

- to improve access to justice
- to reduce the costs of litigation
- to reduce the complexity of the rules
- to remove outmoded and outdated terminology
- to bring consistency to the process.

Lord Woolf's key objective was to ensure that Courts were enabled to deal with cases justly by trying to place the parties on an equal footing, saving expense and dealing with the case in a way proportionate to the amount of money involved, the importance of the case and its complexity. He also wanted to see cases dealt with expeditiously and with an appropriate amount of court time.

In the **legal process** patients will generally instruct a solicitor who specialises in clinical negligence cases. Some claimants bring a case themselves and they are known as '**litigants in person**'. Such people have achieved stunning success because the court may help them to achieve a fair outcome although their inexperience may cause confusion to all involved in the court process and success is certainly not guaranteed.

Legal costs may be considerable in some cases involving osteopaths. The general position in the UK is that the loser in a case pays the costs of the winner. If a claimant discontinues a case once court proceedings have been issued then he or she is also responsible for the opposing osteopath's costs. It is only when a claimant is legally aided that he or she is not generally responsible for the osteopath's costs if unsuccessful.

Legal costs may be substantial, running into many thousands of pounds. Osteopaths must be insured against claims for negligence. The insurer should provide advice and support at an in-house level, should provide legal representation for the osteopath at any court hearing and should deal with all correspondence so that the osteopath is not troubled by direct contact from the claimant's solicitor. The insurer should pay all applicable legal costs and any compensation awarded by a court or agreed in a settlement.

When a claimant sets out to take action against an osteopath, a solicitor is normally instructed. The claimant must decide how the claim will be funded and there are several possibilities:

- *Legal Aid, also known as public funding:* This is now becoming much harder to obtain following recent changes to the rules governing eligibility.
- *Legal expenses insurance:* Many claimants have this sort of insurance as part of their household buildings and contents policies. Such policies pay the costs of an unsuccessful claim.

With both Legal Aid and legal expenses insurance, claimants will not be liable for costs if the case is lost and there is therefore little risk in bringing a claim.

- *Private funding of a claim:* Some claimants fund their own claims but the huge potential costs of significant claims may act as an effective deterrent in such circumstances.
- *Conditional fee agreements:* Also known as 'no win, no fee' agreements, they are backed by insurance policies to pay the legal costs if the case is lost. Furthermore a claimant's solicitor may receive a success fee if the case is

won. The court can order the success fee and the insurance premium to be paid as additional legal costs if the claimant wins the case.

The Process usually starts with the solicitor obtaining details of the proposed claim and the circumstances surrounding the alleged negligence. An investigation is then launched by the solicitor to assess the merits of the allegation. A request will be made to the osteopath for the release of the clinical records. *If you receive such a request then you should notify your insurance medico-legal adviser immediately. He or she will help you to deal with the request.*

Records must be provided within 40 days and there is a standard (small) fee payable for providing them. The solicitor may also seek medical records from the claimant's general practitioner and any hospital involved.

> ✎ The fee for access to the health records is £10.

A request for records does not automatically mean that a negligence claim will follow. In many cases a review of the records may demonstrate that the osteopath operated in a completely appropriate or professional way. The assessment may be made by the solicitor but frequently the opinion of an expert is sought at this stage to review the available information and to evaluate the merits of the case. The initial assessment is vitally important for the funding arrangements. If the report is not supportive of the claimant's contention then the Legal Aid Board or a prospective 'after the event' insurer will not be prepared to fund the case.

If the expert opinion offers a **reasonable prospect of success** the case may proceed to the next stage. A **letter of claim** is sent to the osteopath or to the insurer representing the osteopath if known.

The letter of claim sets out the claimant's case in as much detail as possible. It contains a description of the alleged facts, the main allegations of alleged negligence, a description of the injuries that the claimant suffered, the diagnosis and prognosis with a description of the remedial treatment and any likely residual damage. It also explains the causation (i.e. how the defendant contributed to or caused the injury alleged) and gives details of the damages sought (the financial claim made).

From the letter of claim the osteopath and the insurance advisers should be able to understand the detail of the claim and enable a full investigation so that the osteopath can answer the allegations. Generally the osteopath's advisers will also acquire full copies of all relevant records and any statements necessary to assist in the assessment. The osteopath will be interviewed by claims staff, and possibly a solicitor acting for the insurer and his or her recollections of events carefully questioned.

Assistance may be obtained by engaging an expert to give an initial opinion on the merits of the case. This will enable the insurer to assess whether it is defensible or whether an offer to settle the matter should be negotiated. The insurer will then enter into discussion with the osteopath about the overall impression of the claim and will seek agreement on the subsequent handling.

The civil procedure rules provide for a 90-day period within which the letter of claim should be answered.

Within the letter of claim the claimant may include an **offer to settle** (also known as a **Part 36 offer**). This sets out the amount that he or she would be prepared to accept to settle the claim. This offer has important implications if it is rejected and the case continues but the claim is finally settled for a sum equal to or less than that made in the original offer. In such circumstances the Court would take the view that the initial offer should have been accepted and it will impose a penalty when assessing legal costs at the conclusion of the case.

The osteopath and the defence advisory team have 90 days to consider the letter of claim, to undertake the necessary research and to construct a full response to the issues. It is hoped that, by going through this procedure, the issues will have been identified and the case resolved without the need for costly and often stressful litigation. In general the outcome of the investigations will result in one of the following responses.

- A rebuttal of the allegation.
- An acknowledgement of the injuries and an agreement to settle the claim as made by the claimant.
- Recognition of a degree of culpability and a counter-offer to settle on behalf of the osteopath. For example, the claimant might seek £50,000 and the osteopath offer to settle for £20,000. As with any offer made by the claimant, there would be cost consequences for the claimant if the osteopath's offer was rejected and in the final settlement the same or a lesser amount was accepted.

Limitation is the term used to describe the point beyond which claimants lose the right to issue proceedings. The law as it currently stands sets the limitation period at the third anniversary of the date on which the incident occurred or the third anniversary of the date from which the claimant became aware that an injury had been suffered. In general, for children below the age of 18, they have until they reach 18 plus three years to make a claim. An osteopath may therefore experience a claim many years after the incident occurred.

Experts are employed to evaluate the clinical management of the osteopath and to make an assessment of the claim and decide whether the osteopath's actions constituted negligence. The *Bolam* test really creates the notion of peer review as the means of assessing the osteopath's work.

When a claimant approaches a solicitor, the solicitor may, as part of his review of the claim, seek initial expert opinion, as may the defence insurer when in receipt of the letter of claim. If the claim is disputed, further expert opinion will be required. Both sides may obtain an expert opinion although the court has the power to instruct both sides to use a single expert. The expert will be provided with detailed instructions by the court and they will be made available to both sides.

The expert must be careful to report only within his or her own area of expertise. The expert's duty is to **inform the court** irrespective of who engages his or her services. The opinion should be independent and should not conceal evidence that might assist the other party.

If the case is not resolved at the pre-action stage, then the claimant must decide whether to issue court proceedings. The osteopath's response to the letter of claim will have made clear whether the insurers had decided that there was no claim to answer.

If there is a rebuttal, and the claimant decides to proceed with the claim, then he or she will have to issue a **claim form**. This is an official court document that lays out the detail of the claim and must have with it an expert report substantiating the claim and a schedule giving the details of the damages sought. Once the claim form is issued at a court it must be served on the osteopath within a prescribed time (four months). The osteopath is now referred to as a defendant.

Once the claim form has been served the osteopath has 28 days to serve a defence, which must fully address all the allegations and the issues contained within the claim form. Once the defence is served, the court will send out questionnaires to both parties to enquire about the number of witnesses and experts that they each intend to call. The court will also explore the possibility of a **stay of proceedings**

☢ You can't keep secret some documents and, in a Perry Mason-esque way, announce them at the trial to make the other side's case collapse. Evidence cannot generally be introduced at trial if it has not been exchanged in accordance with court direction. Furthermore, your antics would be looked on very unfavourably by the judge.

to give the parties the opportunity to see whether they can settle the case without recourse to court. Once all the paperwork is complete the judge will consider all the documents and decide how to manage the case.

The Court Track is a term used to describe the route through the court system for any individual case. Essentially, claims worth less than £5,000 go through the **small claims** court, claims worth less than £15,000 and suitable for a one-day hearing go through the **fast track** and all other cases go through the **multi-track route**. The multi-track is the most likely route for osteopath cases. Depending on the value and complexity of the case it may be heard in a High Court rather than a county court.

The judge will schedule a case conference to agree a timetable for the case leading to trial. It will also be used as an opportunity to identify areas of agreement between the parties and therefore limit the areas of dispute. Judges have wide powers in these circumstances and therefore may make a variety of decisions depending on their perspective of the case.

PREPARATION FOR TRIAL

Once the timetable is agreed, both parties must exchange all relevant documents with the other side. These will generally include all clinical records, all correspondence, all statements and any invoices incurred by the patient as part of the costs identified for the special damages claim. This process is designed to ensure that both parties have all the relevant information available to them.

LEGAL PRIVILEGE

Correspondence between a lawyer and his client need not be disclosed to the other side because it attracts legal privilege. This protection extends to the advisers involved in the case.

WITNESS STATEMENTS

These are generally exchanged at the same time by both sides. The statements will have described the events as recollected by the witnesses. They may include not only the osteopath and the claimant but also such people as receptionists, colleagues, relatives of the claimant, GP and hospital staff and anyone else who was involved. At a later stage, both sides exchange expert witness reports. This then enables each side to discover, consider and appreciate the strengths and weaknesses of the other side's arguments. Once these reports have been seen, it is not uncommon for the parties to agree a settlement.

Once proceedings have been issued the defendant can make a **payment into court** additional to any offer to settle made in the letter of response. If the defendant or the advisers decide on this course of action it is paid into the court office. The claimant has 21 days to consider the offer. As with any previous offer, if the claimant refuses the payment as inadequate and the court subsequently awards the same or less in damages there is a considerable penalty in that the claimant would be responsible for paying his and the defendant's legal costs from 21 days after the payment was made. Such a costs penalty may absorb all compensation awarded.

At **trial** the judge, who will not have been involved in previous case management, will not be aware of any payments made into court. There is no jury. The case will be open to the public and to journalists. Cases involving osteopaths, particularly if there is any salacious element, may attract a lot of journalistic interest. Both claimant and defendant will each be represented by a barrister whom they will have met and with whom they will have had a conference previously.

In the United Kingdom judicial system the court procedure is **adversarial**. It can be a most unpleasant experience and everyone giving evidence will experience it. Each witness will be questioned by his or her own barrister and then be cross-examined by the barrister acting for the other

> ☑️ Osteopaths may be asked for a report about a patient and the treatment provided. The solicitor's letter may contain a sentence such as 'No action is contemplated against you in this matter' or 'There is no suggestion that your treatment is under scrutiny'. Osteopaths wonder whether this is an indemnity against ending up in court if it is subsequently decided that the osteopath does have some sort of case to answer.
>
> The answer is that, subject to time limits, the osteopath can be joined later in a legal action if information suggesting negligence comes to light. The solicitor cannot indemnify the osteopath because he or she cannot be sure that more information may not subsequently emerge.
>
> Advice: before agreeing to give a statement, contact your insurance company's medico-legal adviser and obtain advice about what you should say in a statement.

side. A similar process will occur with expert witnesses and other witnesses for both sides. The judge too may ask questions to clarify the facts. At the end of the case the barristers for the claimant and the osteopath (defendant) will make closing speeches.

After everything has been presented the judge will consider all the evidence and give a **judgment**. The judgment may be given orally or in a written judgment some time after the conclusion of the case. If the claimant is successful then the compensation must be paid within a short time. The winner's legal costs are by convention paid by the losing party. However, it is not uncommon for the judge *not* to award costs against a claimant if they lose, presumably because of awareness that the osteopath is defended by an insurance company.

If either party is dissatisfied with the judgment, either party may appeal.

The whole process of a claim is unpleasant and distressing for an osteopath. The insurance adviser should provide support and assistance and is often friend, confidante and ally as well as adviser. Data are very variable but reassuringly about three-quarters of all claims come to nothing and only about 1 in 20 actually finds its way into court.

Examining and Treating the Patient

Compared to examining and treating a patient, all other risks are a walk in the park. Patients present innumerable threats and risks in this respect. Whenever a patient enters your surgery you have no idea whether the subsequent consultation will go well or badly, whether you will make a correct diagnosis or whether an error will haunt you for ages or whether some other event or incident will cause you and the patient distress.

Let us be clear, though. The vast majority of consultations go really well. The outcome is usually satisfied patients and osteopaths whose professional standards are met.

So why include this chapter? Alas, because success is not always the outcome of a consultation. There is no intent in this chapter to tell you how to examine or treat your patients. Your professional skills are a matter for you and GOsC. Its purpose is to draw attention to known risks and pitfalls that have caught osteopaths in the past in the hope that a bell might ring if you find yourself in a similar situation. Prevention, they say, is better than cure, and osteopaths who have found themselves on the wrong side of the GOsC Professional Conduct Committee or a negligence allegation would wholeheartedly agree.

> **Remember: no notes, no defence**
>
> I know it has been said before, but it can't be said too often!

Osteopaths have to act reasonably. That means undertaking the elements of an examination and providing treatment that would be regarded as normal practice by a reasonable body of your ordinarily skilled colleagues. And don't forget that the notes have to show that you did it.

The process of examining and treating a patient has several components and the risks will be considered under the following headings:

- examining the patient
- appearances
- taking the history
- doing the examination
- providing the treatment.

> ☑ Don't omit the medical examination at the expense of the osteopathic examination.

APPEARANCES

Appearances, they say, can be deceptive. But you can learn a lot from appearances. Some errors occur because osteopaths just do not look at their patients and observation should be a key element of examination. In concentrating on osteopathic examination, the osteopath can miss straightforward medical signs. The best examination will integrate the two approaches.

> ☢ Medico-legal reviews indicate that osteopaths may fail to recognise pallor, oedema, signs of cardiac failure and jaundice. In the osteopathic examination omissions include spinal curvature, posture, holding limbs and avoiding weight-bearing.

Medical studies indicate just how important appearance actually is. The information gleaned from a non-physical examination can be divided into what you see and what you hear. The studies suggest that over half of all information is gained from looking at the patient; the way he or she walks, sits down, moves, gesticulates, the body language in general, as well as more general factors such as dress and more specific medical factors such as the presence of peripheral oedema, breathlessness, colour, clubbing, etc. The clues available visually should not be underestimated.

HISTORY

History often provides vital clues that assist in diagnosis and govern the treatments which may be provided. Allegations of negligence not uncommonly arise from failure to take an adequate history. A review of cases suggests that previous malignancy, evidence of osteoporosis and details of therapeutic drug usage may be missed together with symptoms of worsening pain, unremitting pain and night pain.

THE EXAMINATION

The examination builds on the information gleaned in the history
and enables the osteopath to reach a diagnosis. Examination is clearly a
fundamental part of the treatment planning for the patient and it is not part
of the role of this book to describe how to do it. However, allegations of poor
professional standards and negligence indicate that, on occasion, osteopaths
do forget important elements of the examination and this serves to be a
reminder of areas where care is necessary.

- *Examination of the spine:* Most spinal disorders that are missed and which
  subsequently come to the notice of insurers or GOsC could have been
  diagnosed from the history. The age of the patient, activity and restrictions
  and the mechanism of the injury do not raise an adequate degree of
  suspicion in the mind of the osteopath in such cases.
- *Missed fractures are relatively frequent:* Look out for osteoporosis, a history of
  'odd' accidents, compression injuries and sporting accidents. Fracture of
  the fibula may not be spotted – diagnosis may be aided by percussion or
  tuning fork vibration, which is worthwhile if the injury is in the lower leg.
  Scaphoid fractures escape diagnosis every year.
- *Vertebro-basilar insufficiency:* Amongst the most serious clinical omissions is
  failure to recognise or failure to take account of VBI. A failure to recognise
  a compromised vertebral artery system can have catastrophic results.
  There have been hugely expensive cases round the world and some
  cases in the United Kingdom. It is vital to take a history to establish any
  symptoms, such as dizziness, that might be attributable to VBI. Risk
  factors such as atherosclerosis and smoking should be reviewed and
  blood pressure established. Medication with warfarin, steroids or the
  contraceptive pill may be relevant. If you are satisfied that the history
  does not preclude testing, undertake the physical test for VBI. Note the
  period of time for which the rotation is carried out and any symptoms or
  signs that emerge from the test. If you have any doubts **whatsoever** about
  the condition of the arteries do **not** expose yourself to risk by doing any
  treatment that may compromise
  the vessels. You should also consider referral if the patient is
  young.

> Don't forget the chaperone if
> intimate areas are being examined
> or treated.

During the examination it is extremely important to maintain the patient's modesty, allowing the removal of clothing behind a suitable screen and providing a towel or dressing

> ☑ Remember that particular groups present particular problems, for example red-headed people who may be resistant to drugs and anaesthetics.

gown to cover any personal areas. An allegation of voyeurism or worse can damage or destroy a career. Only necessary clothing should be removed, bearing in mind the balance between good access to areas that need examining and the modesty of the patient. Before examination, make sure that you tell the patient what you are going to do with your hands or with any instruments, so that any action you take does not come as a surprise, particularly in an intimate area.

TREATMENT

The whole crux of risk can be focused on clinical treatment. Osteopaths need to be consistently vigilant and to provide those therapies for which they are trained and in which they are competent. All obvious stuff, but if it was that obvious there would not be claims against practitioners. At the risk of repeating messages given elsewhere, do consider the following before or during treatment of the patient:

- Have you obtained consent and given adequate explanation?
- Be careful not to handle the patient roughly.
- Avoid inappropriate comments, particularly at a time when emotional tensions may be running high. Patients may find themselves more undressed for longer periods than patients of other healthcare professionals.
- Do not fail to assess the reactivity of the patient.
- Do not ignore feedback from the patient regarding treatment.
- Remember to re-assess treatment. You should be careful not to continue with a treatment without critical review. In such circumstances damage may ensue.
- Avoid mechanistic management.
- **Do not take inappropriate risks.** You should not go home at the end of the day wondering whether any of the treatment that you provided was either not correct or not safe.

This chapter is not about how to do a complete examination of a patient. It is about what not to do if you want to avoid trouble. As I said at the beginning of the chapter, the vast majority of consultations and treatments are successful. Osteopathy should be enjoyable as well as a means of earning a living. From a medico-legal point of view, when things go wrong it is often because of saving a few seconds or cutting a corner which exposes the practitioner to needless risk. Being safe is worth the extra minute.

DEALING WITH DIFFICULT PATIENTS

In the vast majority of cases patients' behaviour and attitudes pose no problems, but every practitioner has patients who can be described as *difficult*. Although small in number, they take up a disproportionate amount of time.

They may cause problems in a number of ways:

- They may be rude or aggressive to the osteopath.
- They may be consistently aggressive and demanding to the receptionist but always perfectly charming when they see the osteopath.
- Rarely they may cause actual physical violence.
- They may waste practice time by, for example, failing arranged appointments, etc.
- They may simply have the sort of personality that clashes with the osteopath.

Not every difficult patient presents a problem that is purely vexatious.

- Pain may impair their ability to behave in a socially acceptable manner.
- They may have a mental disorder which modifies their ability to be courteous.
- They may feel aggrieved about previous care (if it failed to bring relief of symptoms).
- The patient may be having a bad day.
- The patient may feel offended or fobbed off by the osteopath or staff.
- The patient may simply be rude or ignorant.

MISSED APPOINTMENTS

Practice efficiency can be disrupted when patients miss appointments without prior notification. If a patient misses an appointment it may be appropriate to write to the person, but before doing so, it is important to:

- establish that the patient did not cancel the appointment – patients get annoyed if wrongly accused of failing to attend
- decide whether it is better to forget it or mention it at a future appointment
- decide whether the patient should be charged or not.

Remember that letters are often seen by people other than the person to whom they were addressed. Ensure the tone strikes the right balance of concern whilst explaining the problems that failure to attend actually causes.

DIFFICULT PATIENTS

Every problem patient presents a unique problem for the practice. Management depends on the nature, frequency and seriousness of the problems that occur. You may consider:

- ignoring a single episode of inappropriate behaviour
- writing to the patient about it
- speaking to the patient about it
- in serious cases, refusing to see the patient for further appointments.

Each of these approaches has advantages and disadvantages. Patients often refuse to accept that their behaviour was in any way difficult, particularly if they did not perceive that it actually was. On occasion rebuking a difficult patient has led to retaliation in the form of a complaint.

1 *Ignore a single incident:* It may be expedient to ignore one incident, especially if the patient is known and the action is out of character. We all have bad days! It is advisable to:
   - note the date and time of the incident and an account of what happened
   - record actual comments if possible

- indicate if any other practice member was present
- decide at subsequent appointments whether to mention it to the patient or simply forget it
- if the patient makes an apology for an outburst, note it in the record. Sadly, apologising is no guarantee that it will not happen again.

2 *Write or speak to the patient:* It may be appropriate to explain to the patient why the behaviour exhibited is not acceptable to you or the practice (e.g. racist comments). If you decide to speak to the patient it is best to avoid an environment where the patient is subjected to a 'dressing down' rather like punishment being meted out to a schoolboy by a headmaster. Discuss the issues of concern in comfortable chairs as equals rather than from behind a desk. Negotiate rather than lecture. If you decide to write to the patient, depending on the events and the subsequent contact with the patient, a letter may be as follows:

Warning about future behaviour

Dear *[name]*

I understand from *[person's name]* that an incident occurred at the practice on *[date]* at *[time]*. It involved *[describe the incident]*.

I would be grateful if you could let me know in writing if my understanding of the sequence of events is in any way incorrect.

The practice provides the highest standards of care for the patients, but we require support and co-operation. We cannot allow incidents of this sort to pass unnoticed and I must inform you that if there is any repetition of this behaviour it may not be possible to provide any further treatment.

The practice is here to assist you and I hope that we can work together in future to meet your expectations of us and our expectations of you.

Yours sincerely,

Mr A N Osteopath

Taking no action

Dear *[name]*

I understand that an incident occurred at the practice on *[date]* at *[time]*.

I have investigated the matter *[and noted your comments]*. I have accordingly decided to take no action on this occasion.

However, I must point out that successful osteopathic care depends on mutual co-operation and I hope we shall be able to enjoy a better professional relationship in future. We are here to help you but we cannot accede to unreasonable demands.

Yours sincerely,

Mr A N Osteopath

There is always a difficult judgement to be made about deciding to take action or ignoring unacceptable episodes and the decision will depend on an array of circumstances. Sometimes it is not appropriate to stir up a hornets' nest but on other occasions ignoring behaviour that is unacceptable may simply result in it being repeated at a later appointment.

The last word on the subject is to contact your professional indemnity insurance medico-legal adviser and discuss the problem before taking action. An independent view may help to resolve or manage the problem.

Consent

Patients have a right to information about their condition. The amount of information with which they are provided will vary according to the nature, severity and complexity of that condition. However, in the United Kingdom any competent adult has the right to give or withhold consent to any examination, investigation or treatment.

Any osteopath who treats a patient without their valid consent may face:

- a criminal action for battery (in England and Wales) or assault (in Scotland)
- a civil action for negligence.

In England and Wales battery is the injuring or even touching of another person deliberately without his or her consent. Therefore battery can lead to a criminal prosecution or a civil claim for compensation. However, an osteopath is most unlikely to be accused of criminal battery because it requires ill intent, which would be very difficult to demonstrate.

There are various types of consent:

- implied, and
- expressed, which may be verbal or written.

You should be careful with implied consent and accept it only for the most basic of procedures. For example, if a patient extends an arm, there is an implied consent that you may examine it visually. To do more requires a more formalised consent, to explain what you intend to do and why.

Many people believe that written consent has greater validity than verbal consent. Under some circumstances this could be true. The signed consent form does indicate that something connected with the consent occurred and the patient signed a piece of paper agreeing to something. However, most consent forms do not detail the areas of the procedure that were discussed and, for that reason, well-written notes explaining the issues considered and written contemporaneously may be at least as valid.

Osteopaths receive guidance about the need for written consent. The GOsC document *Pursuing Excellence* (June 1998) suggests that for the treatment of intimate areas written consent is **advisable** but for vaginal or rectal techniques written consent should **always be obtained**. Osteopaths are strongly advised to comply with the regulatory body requirements.

> **Remember**
>
> No notes, no defence.

Failure to do so will be extremely difficult to defend in the event of a complaint because the GOsC documentation concerning standards and behaviour will be regarded as authoritative guidance with which to be complied and, using the *Bolam* test, the likelihood is that a reasonable body of peers would meet the requirement and obtain written consent.

It is in those circumstances where verbal consent is obtained that good records are vital. As with all questions about the conduct of, or treatment provided by, an osteopath, an allegation may not emerge until months or years after the event. To be asked to recall an incident that happened years previously and to try to establish whether you obtained some sort of valid consent would be impossible without a suitable note in the record.

It is helpful to develop a habit of always writing a note stating that the risks, benefits and alternatives have been discussed. It takes a few seconds and may protect you from days, weeks or years of heartache if a patient accuses you of treatment without consent.

Consent must be **valid**. Sometimes consent is described as informed. In my view, 'informed' is an inappropriate term (although it is popular in the United States) because consent cannot be uninformed. In other words, a patient cannot consent to something that he or she does not understand. However, to be valid requires the osteopath to give the patient enough information to enable them to make an informed decision. The amount of information will vary according to the nature and complexity of the condition requiring treatment or investigation, but it may well include:

- details of diagnosis and prognosis
- uncertainties about diagnosis
- options for treatment
- the purpose of the procedure(s) and the possible consequences
- the benefits and disadvantages
- possible side effects
- the option of not treating the patient and the consequences.

It must also be made clear to patients that they may change their mind at any stage during a course of treatment.

Remember

Consent is a process, not an event.

One of the great difficulties for clinicians of all sorts is that, once convinced that a particular course of treatment will provide benefit for the patient, it is very difficult not to advocate it to the exclusion of any other possible alternatives that the clinician may view less favourably. It does not matter how much better you believe your treatment will make the patient. **If the patient does not consent to it you must not do it.**

Any competent adult can refuse any treatment at any time and, as a professional clinician, you must respect the refusal. In some circumstances patients refuse treatment, usually medical, that will prolong or preserve life. Provided they are competent they have a perfect right to do so.

Clinical point

A well known example of potential 'serious' harm is in the situation where a patient develops unilateral temporary blindness and where multiple sclerosis is the suspected diagnosis. Following resolution there are no further symptoms (40% of patients never develop other features of the disease). It may be considered capable of causing serious harm at a later stage to tell an asymptomatic patient that he or she might have multiple sclerosis.

Some patients are very inquisitive and ask many questions about proposed care. The osteopath really has an obligation to answer all the questions as honestly, fully and objectively as possible. Information can only be withheld from a patient if you believe that the disclosure would cause the patient **serious** harm. Like many things in healthcare, the term 'serious' in not defined in this context and is a matter for the clinician's judgement. However, 'serious' does not mean that the patient would become upset. It implies a much more profound state of distress than that. It is a situation that is unlikely to occur in osteopathy. In all aspects of conduct, the osteopath should keep in mind that he or she should act in a way that is reasonable and defensible. If a complaint about his or her conduct arises subsequently, the onus will be on the osteopath to explain and justify the actions. In the context of consent, the osteopath will need to explain what information was provided and demonstrate that it was adequate.

Wherever possible the osteopath should explain personally to the patient about proposed treatment and obtain the consent himself. The osteopath has the responsibility of ensuring that the consent process is completed satisfactorily. However, the process may be delegated to a suitably trained and qualified colleague who has sufficient knowledge of the procedure, risks and alternatives.

Competence is the central issue in deciding whether a patient can give consent to a procedure. Competence should be assessed by the clinician managing the case. For a patient to be regarded as competent he or she should meet the following criteria:

> ☢ Write copious notes when competence is in doubt. You may have to depend on them if questions arise later.

- understand the nature and purpose of the treatment
- understand the benefits, risks and alternatives to the treatment
- understand the consequences of refusing treatment
- be able to retain the information long enough to make a reasoned decision
- be able to make a free choice (i.e. not act under duress).

> ✎ If there is any doubt an osteopath should refer to the patient's GP for a psychiatric or psychogeriatric review to assess competence.

There may be cases where the osteopath is unable to decide whether a patient is competent. In such situations the patient's general practitioner may be contacted for guidance. Alternatively, a clearer picture may be obtained by seeking the views of friends, relatives or carers (see below). It is sometimes a difficult decision and the osteopath should be careful to document the stages in reaching the conclusion.

A patient may be incompetent, that is, unable to meet the criteria for competence. In the United Kingdom no one can give consent for another adult. The osteopath must **act in the patient's best interests**. In order to make the decision the osteopath should:

- try to ascertain the past wishes of the patient
- try to encourage the person to participate in the decision if possible – in some (particularly elderly) patients there may be a tendency for them to drift in and out of competence; it may require time to establish their true wishes
- consult with friends, relatives and carers and any other appropriate people
- consider the options for treatment with a view to providing the therapy that will achieve the desired result with the minimum of intervention.

CHILDREN

However difficult the process of consent may appear to be for adults, it is much more complicated in some circumstances involving children.

COMPETENT CHILDREN AGED 16 OR OVER

Such children may be regarded as adults for the purposes of consent. The position is enshrined in the Family Law Reform Act (1969) Section 8.1.

> **Thought**
>
> 'Competence' is such a harsh term when applied to anyone, particularly children. It should be used cautiously and terms such as 'learning difficulties' are generally more acceptable.

'The consent of a minor who has attained the age of sixteen years to any surgical, medical or dental treatment which, in the absence of consent, would constitute a trespass to his person, shall be as effective as it would be if he were of full age; and where the minor has by virtue of this section given an effective consent to any treatment it shall not be necessary to obtain any consent for it from his parent or guardian.'

It is important to note that this statute is confined to consent, **not to refusal**, where parents retain residual rights to overrule the refusal of a child to accept a procedure. Of course, the reality of the situation is that, confronted by a burly 17-year-old refusing to have treatment and a mother saying she wants it done, only a foolhardy osteopath would wade in and try to do it. In such circumstances negotiation is the key and it is very unwise to try to force any treatment of any sort on a child who is adamant that he or she does not want it.

INCOMPETENT CHILDREN AGED 16 OR OVER

With respect to consent, these children are covered by common law. Parents can consent for children who are incompetent when aged 16 or 17.

CHILDREN AGED UNDER 16

A child below the age of 16 has the right to make his or her own decision upon sufficient maturity to understand the nature of the matter requiring decision.

THE *GILLICK* CASE

This now famous case concerned the prescription of oral contraceptives to the daughters of Mrs Victoria Gillick without her involvement or consent. She subsequently took legal action against the health authority and the prescribing doctor (*Gillick v West Norfolk and Wisbech Area Health Authority et al [1986]*). In a case that attracted considerable publicity and discussion, the judge decided in favour of the health authority and the doctor and pronounced that the assessment of children below the age of 16 is a matter for the doctor and his clinical judgement, subject to:

- the child understanding the issues surrounding the prescription and use of the drug (i.e. competence)
- the doctor being unable to persuade the child that she should inform her parents
- a judgement that the child was likely to have sexual intercourse in any event
- a concern that, without appropriate contraceptive advice, the child's physical or mental health may suffer
- her best interests being served.

Clearly this judgment related only to a narrow element of medical care but the concept has been rolled out across the whole of healthcare. Therefore if confronted by a child below the age of 16 he or she may be treated by the osteopath if satisfied that the child is competent.

It is important to note that, as with children below 18, the ruling is confined to consent and not to refusal.

In essence, 'Gillick competence' recognises the right of self-determination of young persons. It acknowledges that parental rights over children are dwindling and that they can be overridden. In effect, the rights of parents are now only residual and are wholly extinguished at the age of majority.

In Scotland, the issue of children under 16 consenting to treatment is detailed in the Age of Legal Capacity (Scotland) Act 1991. The Act states:

> 'A person under the age of sixteen years shall have the legal capacity to consent on his own behalf to any surgical, medical or dental procedure or treatment where, in the opinion of a qualified medical practitioner attending him, he is capable of understanding the nature and possible consequences of the procedure or treatment'.

Refusal of treatment by children up to the age of 18 is treated differently. Parents can override a refusal (though not consent). Refusal (and consent) can also be overridden by a court if it is in the patient's best interests. For the osteopath a child refusing treatment clearly raises issues beyond those of obtaining consent from a parent. A young person determined not to accept treatment is effectively untreatable and it is usually very unwise to try to force treatment on an unwilling child. In certain medical circumstances a degree of coercion may be useful where a particular medical treatment is essential and parental consent is obtained, but in osteopathy when negotiation fails it is usually better to accept that treatment will not be possible and to rearrange an appointment.

From a legal point of view there is asymmetry between consent and refusal because a child's consent is enabling (allows the treatment to proceed) but his or her refusal is **not** disabling (because that consent can be exercised by another).

THE POLICE

Because of the confusion that may surround enquiries by the police, it is worth taking a specific look at this area. The police do not have a blanket permission to obtain information about patients. However, there are no hard and fast rules about releasing information and so an osteopath must make a judgement. However, if that judgement is called into question at a later stage he or she may be required to explain and justify his or her actions to GOsC if a patient lodges a complaint about breach of confidentiality. The buck stops with the osteopath who makes the decision!

The following points may be helpful as general guidance if you are confronted by the police:

1 Remember that apparently innocent information like times of appointments or indeed even whether an individual is a patient may, under some circumstances, constitute a breach of confidentiality.

2 If police turn up at a surgery *without a court order* requiring information about a patient, they do not have an automatic right to obtain it. A police uniform does not constitute authority.

3 If they present a court order signed by a Circuit Judge instructing you to release specific information, you **must** comply with the order. Make sure that you keep a fair copy of all the notes with which you part.

4 If police without a court order seek information about an alleged crime, which is of a minor nature, you may not have any obligation to release it without court direction, especially if it is hearsay or from a third party.

5 If police without a court order seek information concerning a serious crime you may feel it appropriate to release it. You should be satisfied that the information being provided by the police is of an adequate standard, and your justification for the release may be that failure to do so may result in another crime being committed, that serious harm may befall individuals or that failure to release the information may result in the suspect evading justice.

6 Reception and other staff should be instructed **never** to release information to the police without the authority of the osteopath except in very exceptional circumstances.

7 If you receive a request for the release of records, always make a detailed note of the request including:
   (a) the nature of the information requested
   (b) the details of the police officer(s) seeking the information
   (c) your decision whether to release it or not
   (d) your reasons for making the judgement.

8 Don't be 'bounced' into releasing information, especially if you do not believe it to be appropriate to do so. If you are unsure, discuss it with your insurance company medico-legal adviser. Don't be intimidated by a tall police officer because he is in uniform, even with the appearance of the good-looking one in *The Bill*.

Consider a few cases.

1 A patient with a painful knee sits down in your consulting room, removes her stocking and turns the knee towards you.

Do you need her consent to *look* at the knee?

2 You examine and formulate a treatment plan for a patient with a painful back. She tells you she wants a particular form of manipulation that 'cured' a friend with a similar problem. You had not considered using the treatment and you are not convinced that it is appropriate in this case.

Do you accede to the patient's wishes?

3 'Doctor, do whatever you need to do to make my back better.'

Is that consent to treatment?

4 A 36-year-old woman with learning disabilities and a mental age of three needs some osteopathic treatment. Her mother, who has brought her to the practice, asks the osteopath to go ahead.

What should the osteopath do?

5 Halfway through treatment for a painful neck, the patient decided that he did not want any more treatment. You remonstrate with him saying that you have nearly finished and it needs just one more manipulation. The man insists that you stop.

Should you?

Answers to these exercises can be found in Appendix 1 (*see* pages 151–2).

After reading about consent you really need one!

CONFIDENTIALITY

We all expect our most personal information to be kept secret. In a world where communications are becoming easier and more information is available to more people it is getting increasingly difficult. However, being an osteopath gives practitioners certain privileges and one of them is that you can ask patients all sorts of personal questions of a confidential nature. What is more, it is reasonable to expect answers and, if the answers are not forthcoming, you have the right to refuse to undertake the treatment. However, the privilege of being able to access confidential information brings with it an ethical obligation to maintain that information confidential.

Confidentiality is a central tenet of the relationship between patient and osteopath, as with all other healthcare professionals. It has been a vital part of the code of medical ethics throughout history. The **Hippocratic Oath** states:

> 'All that may come into my knowledge in the exercise of my profession or in daily commerce with men, which ought not to be spread abroad, I will keep secret and will never reveal.'

The Oath was modified by the **Declaration of Geneva** to read:

> 'I will respect the secrets which are confided in me, even after the patient has died.'

Of course you don't need the pronouncement of a white-haired bearded old Greek or a bunch of Swiss gnomes to know that everything that you learn in the privacy of the consulting room should be kept confidential.

> ☢ If in doubt, keep it confidential and seek advice from insurance company advisers.

Confidentiality will almost always be **absolute**. It is a key requirement of good practice. If osteopaths did not keep confidential what they learn during

Every osteopath should eat, sleep and read *Pursuing Excellence* every day. Yeah, right! At least I've said it.

the course of consultations, they would not attract the confidence of patients. Patients would not want to release information for fear that it might be transmitted to others. Release of inappropriate information could lead to stigmatisation and discrimination. In keeping such information from the healthcare professional, their own treatment might be compromised if a decision on management were to be made in the absence of key relevant detail. Worse still, a patient in need of treatment might decide not to attend an osteopath altogether if he or she felt that there was a significant risk of breach of confidence. Confidentiality is a cornerstone of trust and good practice.

The General Osteopathic Council takes a firm view on confidentiality. In a series of sections in the document *Pursuing Excellence* it outlines the ethical duties of an osteopath. Every osteopath should know the document like the back of their hand.

☺

6 Here are some other conundrums:

- If a schoolteacher asks whether a child has come for treatment at a certain time, should you confirm it?
- If the police ask you about a patient attendance should you tell them?
- If a husband telephones and asks about his wife's treatment, should you say?

For answers *see* page 152.

Of course, during the course of a consultation there will often be a barrage of information being made available. Is it all confidential? Is it reasonable, for instance, to tell a husband, if he rings the surgery, that his wife has come in for osteopathic treatment, or is such information confidential?

Aside from any ethical or legal considerations, it is important to consider the release of information from the patient's perspective. If it were your information would you want it to be released to other people without your consent? It is a highly emotional question but, fortunately, the law provides many of the answers for what constitutes confidential information.

Several court cases have established a **legal duty of confidence**. As with many legal diktats, the elements expounded are really back-to-front and describe those characteristics of information that enable a breach:

- Information must have the necessary quality of confidence.

- Information must be disclosed in circumstances implying an obligation of confidence.
- Unauthorised disclosure would cause harm to the confider.
- The disclosure itself would have the potential to harm the patient in the future.

In essence these criteria make clear that information provided in the privacy of a consulting room must be regarded as confidential. The consulting room environment certainly implies an obligation of confidence and any disclosure of information would be a breach of the obligation, whether or not any actual harm had occurred.

> ☑ Staff training is vital and the confidentiality message should be reinforced on a regular basis.

It is important to remember that the duty of confidentiality extends to the members of the practice team. As an osteopath you have a legal responsibility for members of your team. Do you know what your receptionist is saying when you are not there? Breaches of confidentiality by staff would be a serious disciplinary matter.

Sometimes patients bring with them family members or friends to act as a chaperone or merely to provide some moral support. Osteopaths should be very cautious about what is said in the presence of others. If, for example, a young woman patient was consulting about a painful shoulder, with her mother in attendance, it would be wholly inappropriate to release information, for example, about her medical history. If it became necessary, for instance, to confirm that the woman was still taking an oral contraceptive pill, it would be necessary to find a way of asking the question at a time when the patient was alone. Furthermore, osteopaths should be very careful about answering even apparently innocent questions posed by relatives during the course of a consultation.

Of course, over time, relationships (professional!) develop between practitioners and their clients, especially in osteopathy where the physical interaction may be very close. Sometimes it is very difficult to keep confidential information concerning third parties about which you may be asked. Rather than a brusque 'I cannot tell you', developing a stock phrase such as 'Unfortunately my professional code prevents me from telling you' sounds less like telling them to mind their own business.

As with consent, children provide a special problem for the osteopath. The age at which a child will be able to consent to treatment, i.e. becomes competent to make the decision, will vary according to the degree of judgement and maturity that the child can apply. In reality the osteopath should be able to discuss confidential medical matters with the parents of any child who is not considered competent to make his or her own decisions. Once they are competent, at whatever age, they acquire the right to confidentiality enshrined in the *Gillick* judgment.

The same situation applies with patients who are mentally disadvantaged. If the patient has, in the opinion of the clinician, a sufficient level of understanding then they have the right to consent and therefore the right to retain control over disclosure of their own records.

There are certain circumstances where disclosure of patient information may be considered justified. **Justified disclosure** is relatively rare and in the vast majority of circumstances absolute confidentiality should apply. Clearly the information imparted to the osteopath belongs to the patient and the patient normally has the right to choose when and to whom he or she wishes to impart that information.

In some circumstances the patient will consent to the osteopath releasing information that would normally be regarded as confidential to third parties. Such third parties might include:

- other healthcare professionals to whom the patient is referred or who might be involved in providing care for the patient
- insurance companies seeking information relating to claims for injuries or other matters where the osteopath is in possession of that information
- solicitors acting for the patient or for others.

In certain circumstances disclosure may be justified **without** the patient's consent.

- *Where there is a legal or statutory requirement:*
  - certain Acts of Parliament, for example if a patient is suspected of being a terrorist

☑ In circumstances where data are requested, osteopaths should look carefully at the information provided. If they have any doubt that it is appropriate to supply all the information, they should discuss the matter with the patient and get a signed consent confirming what is to be released. If the patient asks for information to be withheld from a solicitor or insurer for instance, the osteopath should make clear in supplying the data that *some information was being withheld at the request of the patient.* Such a situation might arise for example where a solicitor is reviewing an accident six months earlier but asks for records dating back 20 years. The osteopath may well feel it is wise to enquire of the patient whether he or she wishes to part with all the information to the solicitor.

- serious injury or dangerous occurrence.
- *When ordered to do so by a court:* If the osteopath receives a court order instructing him to release his records, then he must comply with the order. However, if the request comes from a court official or a lawyer without a court order there is no requirement to release the records unless there is another ground. If the records are required by a coroner's officer (police officer) then the osteopath should comply.
- *Where there are medical grounds:* Such a circumstance might be to the relative of a patient with a terminal illness in order to assist the relative in providing the necessary care. This possibility is remote in osteopathy.
- *In the public interest:* Such a situation may occur where there is a substantial risk that failure to disclose information may result in the patient suffering serious

> ☑ If parting with notes to an insurance company or solicitor make sure that there is a recently signed consent covering the whole release.

> ☑ Never part with records without taking a photocopy first.

> ☢ There are two important things to remember when disclosing confidential information.
> 1 Write hugely comprehensive notes. If there is a to-do about the release later, those friendly people at GOsC may ask you to explain and justify your reasons for releasing the information. Woe betide you if you can't remember why you did it!
> 2 Only release information to the appropriate authority. Breaching confidentiality does not mean that you can tell the world and his wife.

harm or death or someone else suffering serious harm or death. The osteopath has to decide whether the duty of care to an individual or to society overrides the duty of confidentiality to the patient.

If you are confronted with a request to breach the confidentiality of a patient there are a number of questions that you should ask in trying to assess whether such a breach would be reasonable.

- What information does the enquirer want to know?
- Why do they want to know it? Is there some other way that they can find out the information without the need for you to breach confidentiality?
- By what authority do they seek it? Do they have a court order or some other authority that gives them a right to the information?

- What grounds can justify the release of the information? An osteopath placed in a situation like this has to recognise that, whatever decision is made, he or she will be very unpopular with someone. In situations where a release is required the osteopath should:
  - have a period of quiet reflection to assist him in deciding what to do
  - contact the medico-legal adviser at the professional indemnity insurance company and discuss the matter.

Remember that patient autonomy is the central feature of confidentiality and is paramount. It is only in a very small number of cases that there is a justification for the release of any confidential information. Breaching confidentiality will cause patients to lose trust and confidence in the profession, resulting in inadequate information or failures to attend for treatment. The information belongs to the patient and the patient will normally always have the right to decide when and if the information is released to someone else.

PATIENT RECORDS AND THE LAW

Osteopaths keep records for their own access to assist then in planning and treating patients and to remind them of treatment previously provided. It is less than 35 years ago that patients were normally prohibited access to their records. However, successive Acts of Parliament have given patients full access and osteopaths should understand what the Acts are and how they should comply.

THE DATA PROTECTION ACT 1984

This was the original Act permitting access to patient information held on computer record. The Act was repealed when the 1998 legislation was enacted.

THE ACCESS TO HEALTH RECORDS ACT 1990

This Act applied to manual records held by the practice. It gave patients the right of access to those records made after 1 November 1991, although the practitioner could release all records if he or she wished to do so. There were certain exemptions which were essentially the same as those incorporated in the Data Protection Act 1998 (see below). The Access to Health Records Act was repealed in respect of living patients when the Data Protection Act 1998 came into force **except for deceased patients**, whose records should still be processed under the provisions of the Act if a request is properly received (i.e. from the next of kin, the executor of the will or anyone who can demonstrate a pecuniary interest in the will).

THE DATA PROTECTION ACT 1998

This Act came into force on 1 March 2000. It repealed the earlier Act of 1984 and its provisions apply only to living individuals. The Act includes all manual health records and all electronic records, whenever they were made.

The Act applies UK-wide.

The Act sets out eight data protection principles. They state that data shall:

- be processed fairly and lawfully
- be obtained only for specified and lawful purposes
- be adequate, relevant and not excessive
- be accurate and kept up to date
- not be kept for longer than necessary
- be processed in accordance with the rights of the data subject
- be held securely
- not be transferred to a country outside the EEA without adequate safeguards.

Health records are any records containing information relating to the physical or mental health of the individual (patient). They may include pictures, diagrams, photographs and video recordings.

Patients may have access to their records under Section 7 of the Act. The request must be made in writing. A standard access fee of £10 is payable for electronic records but rarely a further fee of up to £50 may be charged for very bulky paper records. It has been suggested that 33p per sheet may be a suitable charge for manual records. The Act provides for the documents to be supplied within 40 days.

> ☢ When any documents are destroyed they must be incinerated or shredded with appropriate safeguards for confidentiality throughout the procedure.

The Act provides for the release of **all** records but there are specific exemptions. The data controller (you!) can exclude any information that breaches the confidentiality of a third party (who is not a health professional and who has not consented to the disclosure). Disclosure may also be withheld if its release is likely to 'cause serious harm to the physical or mental health or condition of the data subject (patient) or any other person'. Causing serious harm does not mean that the patient might not like the information much, or indeed may be upset by it. It must cause *serious* harm. This latter restriction is most unlikely to be encountered by an osteopath.

A patient can ask for inaccuracies in their record to be corrected. If dissatisfied they may complain to the Data Protection Commissioner or apply to the court for a court order for compliance. The court could order an osteopath to rectify, block, erase or destroy inaccurate data or require that the record be supplemented with a statement setting out the true facts. Patients can now claim compensation for damage or distress caused by a breach of the Act.

NOTIFICATION

The Act requires that a data controller (that's you!) must provide the Data Protection Commissioner with certain particulars including the name and address, a description of the personal data being processed, the purpose of the processing and a description of the recipients.

Any osteopath receiving a request for notes under the Data Protection Act should immediately contact the medico-legal adviser at the insurer for advice and guidance.

THE ACCESS TO MEDICAL REPORTS ACT 1988

This Act applies to reports supplied for employment or insurance purposes by a practitioner who has been responsible for the clinical care of the individual. If a request for a report is made, the request must be accompanied by a valid signed consent from the patient concerned or the practitioner must seek suitable consent to provide the report. The patient must also be notified that the report has been sought, and that he or she has the right to see the report before it is sent to the employer or insurer if he or she chooses to do so.

If the patient **chooses to see** the report, the employer or insurance company must notify the practitioner about this. If the patient does not arrange access, the practitioner must wait at least 21 days before sending off the report.

If the patient sees the report, he or she may ask the osteopath to amend any part of the report which is considered to be inaccurate. The osteopath may either comply with the patient's wishes or append to the report a statement of the patient's view. The osteopath should have written permission from the patient before sending off the report.

Patients who choose **not** to see the report should sign a statement to this effect. However they may change their mind by writing to the osteopath concerned and may see the report for up to six months afterwards.

OSTEOPATH RECORDS

Everyone knows the jokes about doctors' handwriting. Well, it's not just doctors. But, as Bob Dylan so famously sang, 'The Times They Are A Changin''. A much greater focus is being placed on record keeping and a high standard is now expected.

Many changes may impact on record keeping. Here are just a few of them:

- patients having greater involvement in choices associated with their own care
- increasing patient-centred, rather than task-orientated notes
- patient access to their records
- clinical audit and governance
- the increasing use of computers.

> If it wasn't documented, it wasn't done.

> ☢ Up to 40% of claims for medical negligence may be indefensible because of documentation problems. Make a note of that!

We should first understand what constitutes a record. Well, like Enid Blyton, the records should contain a famous five:

1 Identify the patient.
2 Support the diagnosis by having a clear history and examination.
3 Justify the treatment.
4 Document the course and results and evaluate the outcome.
5 Be prepared to change therapies where effectiveness has not been demonstrated.

> ☑ There is nothing a mischievous barrister likes more than to ask an osteopath to read a completely illegible entry in the notes that may have been written years earlier. It is easy to look *very*, *very* stupid.

It is also nice to have some positive comments. Not essential, but descriptions of positive improvements may well be valuable if everything goes pear-shaped later on.

In general, osteopath records are quite good. However, some are incomplete and quite a lot are illegible.

Remember, the notes may be all you have if a complaint or a claim is made weeks, months or even years later. You can be sure that the patient will be able to describe every last aspect of the treatment down to the length of time of the appointment and the colour of your nail varnish (if you are that way inclined). You, on the other hand, will **only** have your notes and if they do not state your case well enough then you are in the proverbial. Don't forget you charge by the hour (or by the minute in some cases!) and so add a couple of extra minutes to ensure that you do not cut any corners on your record keeping. Legibility should be supported by using black, non-fading ink.

Watch out for the common risks. Here's the Top 10:

Problem	Solution
Identity of patient, especially if two with the same or similar names	Make sure that the notes have a name hazard sticker on them
Ensure that key elements of the past medical history are recorded	A standard checklist may avoid the occasional aberration
Avoid abbreviations that confuse, e.g. PID	Yes, we all know it's Prolapsed Inter-vertebral Disc and not Pelvic Inflammatory Disease, or is it? Be very careful with abbreviations. Either write out terms in full or, if you use abbreviations regularly, provide a key that shows what each one means
Consent	If they agreed to a course of treatment verbally, make a note that they did so and when
Continuity of records	Ensure accuracy and that they clearly indicate progress or deterioration in the condition
Disparaging comments	*Never* use disparaging comments or rude abbreviations. Patients can see their records and they will be infuriated
Audit and research	With increasing requirements for CPD and upcoming appraisal, ensure that notes can be used to extract data if necessary
Delay in writing records	Notes should be contemporaneous, that is, written within 24 hours (certainly no more than 48 hours) after the consultation
Protection	Make sure they protect you and the patient
Security	Make sure they are secure, unavailable to unauthorised persons and protected from damp, infestation, etc. You never know when you might need them!

> ☢ Do not leave spaces in notes that you can fill in later if you need to beef up your records. It used to work quite well but it is no good now. The problem is that ink can be forensically dated – embarrassing if the claimant's lawyer finds a sentence in the middle of the notes that is three years younger than the rest!

ABSENCE OF INFORMATION

Absence of information is of course the key problem with legible and otherwise acceptable information. It is no good professing that your treatments produced a complete cure when the patient alleges in a claim that she cannot do the shopping, carry the children or walk around for more than five minutes. If your contemporaneous notes said that she could walk three miles without pain and had resumed her limbo-dancing career, you will be in a much stronger position. Judges (and other people) are still inclined to believe contemporaneous notes. They were, after all, written before there was any suggestion of a problem in most cases. It is difficult to lie in notes when you don't know how things may turn out in the future.

ALTERATIONS

Never, never, never destroy, alter or re-write a previous record under any circumstances whatsoever, tempting though it may be on some occasions. You are likely to be found out, either by the forensic tests (if the patient or the lawyer suspects that you changed notes in circumstances that they remember differently) or because you make statements that do not accord with the situation at the time. Patients may ask for a copy of their notes and, if you forget and make an 'amendment' it will irreparably damage your credibility if it comes to light – likely if the patient's copy is different to your 'original'.

The other consideration in respect of changing records is that it destroys your integrity and your professionalism.

Finally, if you want to know porridge only as a warming breakfast cereal, **never** change a record.

BIASED NOTES

Biased notes should be avoided. Try to avoid phrases such as 'the patient is always complaining' or 'the patient is too demanding'. It may be absolutely true, but in the wrong place (such as a court) it will put you in a bad light. It is also worth remembering that emotive comments such as 'patient had a good week' tend not to be very helpful. Did the patient have no symptoms, can she walk twice as far, is her pain now more bearable or did she really have a good week and meet Brad Pitt for an exuberant fling? Having a good week has a lot of different meanings and it is worth being explicit.

GOOD QUALITY NOTES

These are what most osteopaths produce. Check yours against the checklist below and be sure that they comply. Good notes equal less risk and less chance of meeting those nice friendly lawyers and judges at the court or at GOsC!

Patient details
Current complaints
History of current complaints
Past medical history
Social history
Examination and findings
Treatment plan
Patient consent
Progress of treatment. Ensure date recorded each time
Measures of improvement or deterioration
Changes of treatment
Patient consent
Dispersal
Referral to specialist/colleague/reason
Discharge – advice given and date
Instructions for return if required

SOME OTHER THOUGHTS ABOUT NOTES

- *How much should you write?* The glib answer is, of course: as much as you need to. Some osteopaths take the view that the records should record all the findings from the history and the examination. Others feel that they should be written on the basis of exception reporting. Experts take the view that both approaches are acceptable but that the parameter for successful notes is not how long they are. Pages of meaningless drivel are valueless if a patient later complains. You need to write sufficient to ensure that you can efficiently assess the patient from the notes at the next appointment, that all key findings are noted and that, should a problem arise months or years later, the notes will support you and enable you to defend, explain and justify your actions and the care you provided.

- *Do you ever wonder why a patient has changed to your practice?* Is it your stunning good looks, your sartorial elegance, your winning smile or your engaging conversation? Or could it be because you are a good osteopath? Is it simply because you are local, easily accessible or have you been highly recommended by other patients? It is well worthwhile trying to establish what may have led to the patient joining the practice. Ask a sensitive question or two. Perhaps there is dissatisfaction with a previous osteopath. What makes him or her think that you can succeed where another osteopath has failed?

  Think about asking:
  - why the patient had changed osteopath
  - what the patient has been told about the current physical state and any diagnoses that have already been made
  - dates of treatment and treatments given
  - what payments were made (but be careful and difficult to discover).

- *What do you do when a patient comes to see you after treatment with another osteopath has been unsuccessful?* This can be very tricky. No one likes to be critical of a fellow professional. Perhaps the patient will ask you what you think about the treatment that has been provided previously. Your primary obligation in such circumstances is to explain **current treatment needs** by assessing the current physical status. The osteopath should recommend treatment. There is no requirement for an osteopath to make a judgement about any suggestion of negligence concerning a previous osteopath.

  Avoid getting drawn into a difficult situation. Don't guess

> ☢ This does not mean you have to be dishonest to a patient to protect a colleague. You have responsibility to the patient and to GOsC not to conceal poor or questionable care. However, that does not mean jumping to conclusions about the circumstances under which particular diagnoses were reached or treatments undertaken.

why an osteopath undertook a particular course of treatment – you were not present at the time of the original history, examination and diagnosis. You cannot tell what signs were present at the time of the original consultation. You should explain that you are not in a position to make a comment on why the previous osteopath treated the patient in a particular way.

Should you need to know about previous treatment for any reason, write to or telephone the osteopath. Do not make 'off the cuff' remarks about particular approaches to treatment. Casual or unguarded remarks may lead to the launch of a complaint against the previous practitioner. It could be your comments that set the whole thing off and you might then become entangled in any subsequent actions and be required to justify your remarks.

Finally: do your records reflect well on you? Make sure you can answer the following questions:

- Do the notes tell you everything you need to know about the patient's condition?
- If another osteopath needed to treat your patient using your notes, would they be legible and comprehensible?
- If the notes were all you had to defend a claim from several years earlier, would they be adequate?
- If your reputation depended on your notes, would you be OK?

Think about it.

- *How long should you keep records?* It is surprising that opinions vary on the need to keep records. Below is some guidance on what might be appropriate.
  - The time limit set for initiating litigation under the Civil Procedure Rules is three years from the date of the incident or (and here's the rub) three years from when the patient becomes aware of the incident. Generally the latter situation is relatively unusual for osteopaths, but occasionally a case may come to light 5, 10 or more years after the event.
  - If a patient is under 18 then the records should be kept as a minimum until the patient reaches eighteen years of age plus three years.
  - Records for patients in HM armed forces should not be destroyed.
  - Records for those serving a prison sentence should not be destroyed.

The best advice is to keep the records for as long as possible, bearing in mind the minimum guidelines above, and, when you can't move for records, destroy the oldest first after the special groups have been identified.

PERSONAL RELATIONSHIPS WITH PATIENTS

The healthcare professions provide a unique window on the distress and suffering of patients and osteopaths develop a close physical and personal relationship with their clients. Patients often return to see the osteopath many times and they see him or her not only as an expert in treating their symptoms, but also as someone in whom they can confide their anxieties and thoughts. In consequence patients often see their osteopath as their friend, and the relationship is often reciprocated. There is nothing unprofessional in such a relationship and there is no reason why an osteopath cannot continue to treat a patient who is regarded as a friend and, indeed they may meet socially.

Such a relationship does, however, bring with it inherent potential dangers for the osteopath. It is sometimes difficult to ensure that the relationship is a purely social one and that it should have no influence on professional opinion. The GOsC document *Pursuing Excellence* makes clear that the role of patient and that of friend should be kept clearly separated.

Of course a much greater problem emerges when an osteopath and a patient form an emotional or a sexual relationship. Every practitioner knows and understands the problems that this causes and some osteopaths have suffered at the hands of patients who have 'blown the whistle', usually when such a relationship comes to an end. Again, the GOsC guidance is quite clear and emphasises that it is a professional duty of the osteopath absolutely to avoid placing him or herself in such a position, and also to avoid any behaviour that might be construed as in any way inappropriate.

> **Shakespeare knew**
>
> Scrutiny of GOsC cases shows the validity of:
> ___
>
> 'Heaven hath no rage like love to hatred turn'd nor Hell hath no fury like a woman scorned'
>
> *The Taming of the Shrew*

All professional bodies offer similar advice in such circumstances. They instruct that any practitioner who finds that he or she is becoming emotionally or sexually involved with a patient *must* end the professional relationship immediately. The patient must be treated by another osteopath.

Inevitably, emotional and physical relationships will develop between osteopath and patient on occasion. If it is discovered and reported to the Council, there will be a hearing of the Professional Conduct Committee. The penalty handed down by the PCC could be very harsh depending on the circumstances of the case. It is common to hear criticism and disapproval of any osteopath who finds him or herself in such a situation.

It is usually a male osteopath and a female patient. It should be remembered, however, that the circumstances in which such relationships develop are often complex and the emotional distress and damage to other personal and professional relationships so great that osteopaths finding themselves in such situations need support and a sympathetic ear rather than criticism. It often falls to the insurer's medico-legal adviser to provide that support and assistance.

Sometimes an osteopath will become aware of advances made by a patient. In such circumstances the osteopath should not make light of it or ignore it. He or she should take definitive action in the event that the patient makes an inappropriate comment or action. It may be best to make a clear statement to the patient warning them that such a comment or action is unacceptable or, if serious, advising them that they should find another osteopath. In such circumstances a proportion of patients will be apologetic or claim that the comment or action was misunderstood.

If the osteopath does decide to continue to treat the patient it should be made entirely clear that if there is any repetition of the behaviour the professional relationship with the patient will be terminated immediately. A comprehensive note should be placed in the patient record describing the nature of the inappropriate behaviour, the warning given to the patient and the ultimatum about any further misbehaviour.

Sometimes it is easier to write to a patient after he or she has left the surgery. The letter might say something like:

> 'In the surgery today you made comments (did something) that I found wholly unacceptable. Your advance was neither solicited nor acceptable. In order for us to have a professional working relationship and for me to continue providing your osteopathic treatment I must emphasise that you must not behave in any way inappropriately. Our relationship must remain entirely professional. If you make any further advance I shall have no alternative but to terminate the care that I provide for you.'

It is important to remain firm and resolute, to ensure that all interactions are carefully recorded and to notify any professional colleagues in the practice of the events in case you need to seek their help, for example by transferring the patient to them.

WHISTLE BLOWING

'Whistle blowing' is a horrible term. It conjures up unpleasantness and, however professional the osteopath may be, the idea of 'grassing' on a colleague, however poor the quality of his or her work may be, is anathema and feels more at home in an episode of *The Bill*. The feeling of 'there but for the grace of God go I' is strong in respect of professional work and, as poor practice is often (though by no means exclusively) associated with older practitioners, younger colleagues are disinclined to report any shortcomings simply because they know that they will be older one day and threatening a practitioner's livelihood by preventing them from practising seems draconian.

OK, so that's the downside, but there are reasons why it is necessary to consider action.

- An osteopath whose standard of practice is poor may well injure a patient. Supporting a colleague is fine but it should not be at the expense of the wellbeing of patients. The reputation of the whole profession may be damaged by a practitioner whose treatment is hazardous.
- Professional indemnity costs are based on the number and value of claims made against osteopaths. If sub-standard practitioners making mistakes are sued, the costs associated with their lack of competence will have to be spread across all practitioners, the vast majority of whom are of the highest calibre.
- An osteopath knowing that a fellow practitioner is providing a poor standard of practice and putting patients at risk exposes him or herself to risk. If it is discovered that an osteopath has practised whilst unfit or inadequately skilled to do so, and it comes to light that you knew, **you may well find yourself in front of the General Osteopathic Council.** The punishment for knowingly ignoring poor practice may be as harsh as that applied to the practitioner whose standards are in question.

Of course, if you become aware that a colleague is performing badly, he or she may be in desperate need of help. What should be done to help? It really all depends on your relationship with the practitioner in question. You might consider:

- *Talking to the practitioner yourself:* If you do, there is a risk that you will be confronted with an aggressive response and a non-preparedness to discuss any problems at all. You could also find yourself in a difficult position if he or she seeks your help and places you in a position where you effectively have to monitor subsequent work. Not a good plan!
- *Involving a senior colleague if one is available:* Sometimes when confronted by a peer in age and seniority the practitioner will admit to the problems.
- *Contacting your defence insurer and seeking advice:* Sometimes having someone independent with whom to discuss the matter is very helpful.
- *Reporting the osteopath to the General Osteopathic Council.*

In some cases poor practice is the result of physical illness or emotional or psychiatric disorders. In such cases it is very important to ensure that the practitioner receives help quickly. The Health Committee of the General Osteopathic Council is supportive and their objective is always to help the osteopath to recover wherever possible and to facilitate and expedite a return to practice.

At the end of the day you will have to wrestle with your conscience if you become aware of a poorly performing colleague. However, if you do nothing it could lead to damage to patients, financial and professional damage to you and your colleagues, and you may end up before the beak! It really isn't worth it.

CHAPERONES

During the course of many osteopathic procedures patients may be required to remove clothing and submit themselves to intimate examinations. Many treatments involve a physical closeness on the part of the osteopath. In such circumstances, where treatment is provided perfectly properly and to the highest standards, nonetheless it may be open to being misconstrued. For that reason, healthcare professionals in general are moving towards having chaperones available for their own protection and for the reassurance of patients during any examination that is of a personal nature.

Many practitioners are still opposed to the practice, fearing that privacy is lost, that there are difficulties in finding suitable chaperones and that the cost of doing so may be considerable. However, the more general view is that chaperones are valuable in a number of situations or combinations of situations:

- where the patient is of the opposite sex to the osteopath (allegations involving same-sex inappropriate behaviour are very rare)
- where clothing is removed and particularly where the more personal areas of the body may be partly or wholly exposed
- where treatment involves close physical contact
- where a patient asks for a chaperone
- where the osteopath feels that his or her own safety may be compromised without a chaperone.

Publicity about chaperones may be done by having a notice in the waiting area stating that arrangements can be made for a chaperone to be in attendance on request. In addition, a similar notification can be placed in the practice booklet.

Sources of chaperones may either be members of staff (in circumstances where there are suitable staff that are available for such duties) or friends or relatives of the patient. There has been discussion about:

- whether the chaperone should be able to see what is being done or whether it is adequate simply to hear any exchanges between patient and clinician
- whether a chaperone should be in the room in which the treatment is being provided or whether an open consulting room door and a receptionist sitting in a nearby (say) waiting area is adequate.

Opinions vary on these issues. It is the opinion of the author that, in the current climate, it is adequate for a chaperone, when required, to be in the same room as the patient and osteopath but separated from them by (say) a curtain so that it is possible only to hear rather than see what is happening. It seems extremely unlikely that, if an osteopath were to act in an unprofessional manner, the patient would not make some sort of comment that would be audible to the chaperone. The chaperone is present not to 'catch the osteopath out' but for reassurance. If the patient requests that the chaperone observes what is being done the osteopath would normally accede to such a request, though the chaperone might be placed in a position where the view was general rather than specific, particularly when intimate areas are being examined. It might be adequate for a chaperone (receptionist) to be in an adjacent room but, for the chaperoning to have validity, the receptionist should be able to clearly hear what is being said.

Staff should fully understand the need for confidentiality of the same standards as that applied by the osteopath. The whole practice team has a duty of confidentiality. However, the use of relatives or friends does pose a problem of confidentiality. For example, if a patient attends an osteopath for treatment for a back problem, the agreement of the patient for the friend or relative to act as chaperone should only be assumed to be for the specific treatment for which consent has been given. The osteopath in that example should not discuss medication or previous gynaecological history or issues surrounding other family members in the presence of the chaperone. Such a conversation should occur at the beginning or end of treatment, before there is any proximity between client and osteopath, and before the chaperone enters the room (or after he or she has left).

> Can I film proceedings and use it as evidence in the event of an allegation of misconduct?
> The idea of producing such videos brings with it a whole new range of risks. Short answer: *no!*

CONSENT

Under normal circumstances if an osteopath offers a patient a chaperone and it is refused, the osteopath should make a clear note of the refusal in the record. If an osteopath wishes a chaperone to be present for his or her own reassurance, then the patient must consent. If the patient refuses consent in circumstances where an osteopath has concerns, the practitioner should consider whether he or she should continue with the treatment unchaperoned.

A chaperone may be of either sex. If the patient brings a friend or relative, clearly their choice will lead to a presumption of acceptability and they should then indicate if there are any circumstances where their chaperone should not be admitted. For the osteopath, it is acceptable to offer a chaperone of either sex (which could, for example, be another osteopath). The patient would, of course, have the right to reject a particular person as unacceptable.

Although chaperones serve to provide reassurance and support for patients they are very important in some circumstances for the safety of the osteopath. A career can be placed in jeopardy by an allegation of unprofessional treatment and, although the idea of chaperones has not been popular with some practitioners, they can provide a crucial level of safety in some cases. The other orthodox healthcare professions all have to address the same issue and it is likely that chaperones will soon be the rule rather than the exception. An osteopath should not be afraid to refuse treatment if he or she feels vulnerable with a particular patient and there is no chaperone available.

DOMICILIARY VISITING

Some osteopaths do domiciliary visiting. It has its advantages. It provides a service that patients might otherwise be unable to access, it provides a degree of flexibility that would otherwise be denied to osteopath and patients and, presumably, it earns a lot of dosh. However, there are possible hazards and the osteopath should consider them if he or she is happy to do such work.

The greatest hazard is of course the risk of exposure to allegations of inappropriate behaviour occurring in the patient's home. GPs have been exposed to this risk since time immemorial and on occasion have fallen foul of serious allegations. Though it is difficult to avoid all risks it is possible to minimise them using a simple checklist of considerations before deciding to proceed:

1 Do you know the patient seeking the visit? If it is a long-standing patient, you know him or her well and you are content that it is safe to go, there is probably no problem. You may not want to attend the home of a new patient on your own.
2 Have you done a visit before? If the request is part of an ongoing treatment, the visit will probably be safer.
3 Have you got any reason to be concerned about the visit? Concerns may exist because the patient has been 'flirty' in the past, or because you will find yourself alone with a patient in circumstances where, following any subsequent allegation, everyone says that it was obvious that you were taking a risk.
4 Are there any alarm bells ringing? Never ignore your own sixth sense. If you think it is a risk, don't do it!

So, what do you do if you decide to do a domiciliary visit and you find yourself alone in a house with a patient who is naked and lying in bed and giving you the 'come on'? The answer is that you should have done and should do the following:

1 If you get a request for a home visit and you decide to go, make sure that the **request is documented** and that your staff member(s) **know that the request was made.**

> ☑ Don't forget that contemporaneous notes are still regarded as a good basis for defence. Always write extra notes in any situation where there may be concerns.

2 If you are visiting a house where there is the remotest possibility that you could be compromised, tell the patient that you want him or her to have a relative, neighbour or friend present as a chaperone. It is reasonable to say that you cannot visit without such a prior arrangement. If you get to the house and there is no chaperone, you should leave at once, making a note of all the events.
3 You can take your own chaperone if you have someone available.
4 If you find yourself in a house, on your own, with a patient who shows any signs of misbehaviour, stop immediately, leave and make detailed notes of what happened and what you did when the patient behaved inappropriately.
5 Finally, *if in doubt, don't.*

MANAGING PATIENT EXPECTATIONS

In the words of Charles Dickens, patients have *Great Expectations*. Over the last two decades we have moved into a seven-day-a-week, 24-hour-a-day, 'I need it now' type of culture where patients who develop acute symptoms have clear expectations of what they want and when they want it. It is often a cause of considerable problems for osteopaths when patients believe that they can offer treatments or achieve outcomes that are not possible, not only for the osteopaths, but for any healthcare professional.

Misleading articles in magazines or by word of mouth may have led the patient to believe that a particular form of treatment is available or likely to be successful when it may be completely inappropriate for their own osteopathic problem. Osteopaths should not assume that patients understand significant amounts about osteopathy. It is frequently the case that even simple procedures are not understood or are misunderstood by patients seeking osteopathic treatment.

Increasing expectations are not confined to the clinical area. They include availability of parking, the comfort and privacy of the waiting area, the expectation of confidentiality when dealing with the receptionist and the level of courtesy and friendliness afforded to them by the osteopath himself as well as by any staff.

> ☢ Complaints and claims frequently arise because the osteopath fails to meet expectations. The description of diagnosis and treatment must be made absolutely explicit at the first consultation.

> ☑ If, at the outset, it is obvious that the patient has expectations you cannot meet, tell the patient, shake hands and let them go with no charge.

A number of common problems arise within the 'expectation zone':

- Treatment of a nature or complexity that is beyond the osteopath.
- A request for treatment in such a way or in a particular sequence that the osteopath does not feel is clinically acceptable or reasonable.
- A patient seeking appointment times that are unavailable, e.g. Saturday afternoons.
- Circumstances where the patient appears rude, aggressive or generally unpleasant or is simply someone that the osteopath really does not want to treat.

Furthermore, those practice policies that will impinge upon the patient's treatment should be made clear. These include:

- arrangements for payment
- arrangements for making and cancelling appointments
- information about the necessary duration of appointments
- expectations when appropriate about what will be accomplished at each appointment.

Whatever it is, *'tell it early and tell it often'*. Perception is everything. How you see it may not be how the patient sees it.
  Look at it this way:

Osteopath	Patient
Reasonable clinical standard	Does it match expectations?
Reasonable outcome	How long will it take?
Prompt and complete payment	How much will it cost?
Quality treatment	Will it hurt?
Notification of any standards that cannot be met	Will I be cured?

Matching what the osteopath can deliver against what the patient hopes for is the trick to ensure a minimum risk of disappointment, failure, refusal to pay and possible litigation.
  The state of the practice is also a potent generator of expectation and the right premises can be reassuring for the patient:

- Are the premises well maintained?
- Are waiting area seats adequate?
- Are the magazines in good condition and recently published?

- Is there adequate facility for privacy and confidentiality?
- Are the toilet facilities adequate and of a good quality?
- Are the consulting rooms efficient and comfortable looking?
- Are there facilities to notify patients of delay in appointments?
- Are brochures available for patients? Are they well presented and do they include information about:
  - the practice
  - telephone numbers
  - the osteopath(s) and staff
  - the types of services that are provided
  - any specialist services or services outside osteopathy, e.g. acupuncture, naturopathy, nutrition
  - public transport and parking arrangements
  - the provision of care in an emergency
  - treatment exclusions
  - the policy (if any) if an appointment is missed or cancelled without adequate warning?

STAFF

Staff are the shop window of the practice. You should consider carefully whether the staff are your best advocate or driving patients away. It is exceedingly difficult to smile continuously and be permanently pleasant, particularly if it is the end of a long day or there is trouble at home. Be there to support staff, to help them to get through those difficult days (and incidentally they may have a lot more trouble with difficult patients than you do) and to meet their training needs. Find out whether the receptionist:

- acts courteously and with a friendly manner
- is able to act as a patient friend, adviser and supporter
- is able to act as an ambassador for the practice
- is able to negotiate and to have management skills
- is good on the telephone
- dresses in a professional manner, clean and smart.

All obvious and basic? Yes, of course they are, but no receptionist will be rude or off-hand to the osteopath. Sometimes they are not so nice and lovely to the patients. See for yourself. Take 30p out of the petty cash, walk down the road to the call box and phone your practice. See how helpful your receptionist is. You might just get a surprise.

Can your staff defuse complaints quickly? All the evidence is that if a complaint is handled quickly and professionally it is unlikely to escalate. Does your receptionist know what to do? Can they avoid disturbance and upset to other patients who might be present? Perhaps some training is necessary?

BAD DEBTS

Bad debts may be a problem for you. If they are, do you have a policy for managing them? Issues will include:

- Is the sum outstanding actually worth claiming for the hassle involved?
- Is it substantial? If the patient refuses to pay, are you ready for a fight?

> **Remember**
>
> Make it easy to pay and you'll probably get paid.

- If a patient doesn't pay, is it because they perceive the treatment to be unsuccessful or of an inadequate standard? Are you certain that you should try to recover the sum?

It is very important that each case is managed on its merits. Negotiation and personal conversation are easy to do and may help you get to the root of a problem if there is one. The small claims court is there as well and should not be ignored. It is cheap and easy to use.

PATIENT SURVEYS

Your services are excellent. They are universally popular and they meet all your patient needs. You know that, don't you? Oh really? Perhaps you should consider a patient questionnaire. They are occurring all through healthcare and they are not all complete rubbish. Sometimes important changes occur because of patient observations that even you may not have thought of. If you decide to try one, make sure you include the following issues:

- a review of services provided
- the opportunity for patients to comment on services they might like to see
- the costs of treatment

- the attitude of the osteopath and any staff
- the ways the practice could be improved.

Expectation is difficult to manage but with a little effort it can reap considerable rewards, avoid disappointment and keep stress levels down for you and the patients.

GETTING TO GRIPS WITH COMMUNICATION

I wonder how many of you remember what three-and-fourpence was? Actually it is nearly 17p in decimal coinage. Somehow three-and-fourpence had a charm and individuality that we have lost. But I digress.

Apparently during a First World War campaign a beleaguered group of luckless soldiers were dug in, with the enemy all around. The commander saw that his only way to survive was to advance but he needed more troops to do it. So he sent a messenger to return as quickly as he could to the headquarters with the message, 'Send reinforcements, I'm going to advance.' The message relay arrangements resulted in the message being passed by word of mouth from messenger to messenger. When the message finally arrived at the Brigade Headquarters the final messenger was able to pass on the information to the Commanding Officer, 'Send three-and-fourpence, I'm going to a dance.'

Silly, yes, but it illustrates how easily communications can let us down and how easy it is for comments to be misunderstood. Get the communication right and the chances are you will get the diagnosis right and the patient will go home reassured, understanding what he or she will have to do and knowing what to expect. It is important to understand that breakdowns in communication are at the heart of most claims for negligence against healthcare professionals.

Communication is, after all, two-way. There is the information that the patient

---

Consider the communications in our own practice – between you and the patient, the patient and you, you and colleagues and you and staff. Any problems?

passes to the osteopath and the information that the osteopath passes to the patient, with quite a lot of chat in the middle. Accuracy is often the casualty of professional conversation and there is a world of difference between, for example, an acute pain and a chronic pain. Yet patients commonly mix the two words and the outcome could be an entirely wrong understanding on the part of the osteopath.

The following suggestions may help you improve communication. Better communication equals lower risk. It has got to be good.

- Let the patient make the initial running. Allow them to voice their concerns and explain their problems.
- Listen with genuine interest. Don't hold the pen, write notes or type onto the computer screen whilst they are talking to you. Concentrating on what is being told to you works wonders.
- Shut up. A study showed that doctors are completely unable (most of the time) to keep quiet for more than 13 seconds. They have an overwhelming need to interrupt patients. I am sure that some osteopaths are as bad, wanting to finish the patients' sentences for them. If a silence develops whilst the patient is talking, keep quiet. The patient may often fill the gap with something more useful or with greater clarity.
- Look for clues as the patient speaks to you:
  - Do they make eye contact?
  - Do they look anxious, sad or angry?
  - What is their breathing telling you?
  - Look at the facial expression and gestures.
  - Does their clothing tell you anything (other than how much you can charge!)?
- Don't rush to judgement. Be prepared to challenge your initial conclusions.
- Ask yourself key questions:
  - What is the key problem that the patient is telling me about?
  - Why this patient?
  - Why at this time?
  Repeat back what they have said to you. This lets the patient correct anything that you may have got wrong or they haven't explained very well.
- Avoid techno-speak and jargon. Even simple words may be misunderstood by bright people.
- Remember that you have a special place in the community. In the minds of many people you are a powerful figure. Don't sit behind a desk and surround yourself with medical equipment, books, papers, etc.

- Make it easy for the patient. Think about their lifestyle, intelligence and resources.
- Remember: perception is everything.
- Look for 'non-verbal leakage' (what a terrible expression). The phrase indicates the need to spot the difference between what the patient says and what their non-verbal behaviour is telling you. Everyone has had a patient who says 'No I'm not depressed' whilst sitting, shoulders slumped, with a sad fixed expression and exuding gloom.
- Consider what your words will mean to the patient. 'Won't' means 'might', 'can't' means 'could' and 'shouldn't' means 'probably will'.
- It is sometimes helpful to speak in the plural to emphasise the 'we're all in this together' approach. Useful words are 'we', 'us' and 'together'.
- Have good leaflets to market, promote, explain and support what you have said. After outlining a series of exercises a leaflet that emphasises what you have said is a great back-up. They should be neat, coloured if the exchequer will run to it, and written in friendly English – not tatty little photocopies.

Leaflets can make a big difference to a practice for the reasons listed above. If you give every new patient a leaflet about the practice (who you are, your qualifications, the practice facilities, staff, opening hours, charges, etc.) the likelihood is that it will be kept next to the telephone, where it will be a constant advert for anyone making a call. Leaflets about particular medical conditions are also useful and, again, provide excellent advertising. The General Osteopathic Council produces a range of leaflets and fact sheets, which include:

- osteopathy and back pain
- osteopathy and pain relief
- osteopathy and work strain
- osteopathy and driving
- osteopathy and arthritis
- osteopathy and pregnancy
- osteopathy for babies and children
- osteopathy and sports
- osteopathy and choosing a bed.

It may be appropriate to use these leaflets as the basis for your own, incorporating into them your own services and some practice details. They need not cost a fortune, with desktop publishing so good these days. What you really need is a 10-year-old who is a computer wizard. He will do everything for you!

If you have practice staff, or you work with colleagues or practitioners from other disciplines, have you looked at communication with them?

- How do you pass information? Not those dreadful post-it notes stuck on windows and computer screens. There have been disasters when they have become detached and lost and messages have not reached the intended recipient.
- Do you actually have a strategy for ensuring relevant information is passed around?
- Do you know what should be passed and what you will say when it is?
- What is likely to go wrong?
- Will a good communication system cost money?
- How will you know if it has worked?

Let's face it. Some osteopaths are really good at communicating with patients and others are, well, less good. Some are attentive, considerate and supportive, whilst others are arrogant, self-opinionated and directive. The latter group includes the 'osteopath knows best' group and they are much more likely to have a clinical negligence catastrophe. They will also damage their own reputations with their clients.

It's a bit of a radical idea but it may be a good idea to create a **patient participation group**. Before dismissing the idea out of hand, the benefits should be considered:

- They will give you feedback on the services you provide.
- They will help you if you have difficulties with other clients or the local authorities.
- They will even fund-raise for you if you want particular bits of equipment.
- They can publicise you in a way you can't and can help to build your practice.
- They will be your best allies if the going gets tough.

So communication is very important, between you and the patients, between you and the community, between you and the staff or colleagues, and between you and the defence insurer, which should be there to give you advice whenever you need it. Most of all, good communication may keep you out of the court or a GOsC hearing. It is worth the effort.

> If you have a really good consultation with a patient who is absolutely thrilled with your care, it is probable that he or she will tell *one* other person, probably a relative. If the consultation is awful he or she will tell *ten* other people. Reputations spread, but the speed is up to you. In this case, bad news travels fast and slow is beautiful!

INFORMATION TECHNOLOGY AND RISK MANAGEMENT

Judging by the records that I see during the course of my medical defence work, most osteopaths still practise in an environment which, in information technology terms, is somewhere between Jurassic Park and the Bronze Age. I rarely see a computerised record.

Handwritten records have their advantages. They are not constrained by the limitations of any system. They tend to be written during a consultation whilst computerised records tend to be written after a consultation. You don't ever see ridiculous entries like 'Miscellaneous disease – other', which one doctor's computer system generates if there is no option to fit what the patient is actually suffering from. However, handwritten notes are not good for audit or research. To be able to press a button and identify how many left-handed, aboriginal men have occupational backache at your practice can be useful and time saving if you happen to want to do it. And believe me (and I am prepared to have actual money with anyone who cares to bet!) the time will come when demographic information is required from every practitioner, just like it is from every doctor now.

GPs are required to use a coding system to record the diseases and disorders that they identify. The coding system does at least give a clue to incidence but some of the codes are truly bizarre. I bet not many doctors use the code for 'Struck by a falling astronaut'. The time will come when all osteopaths have a similar system.

Modern Windows® systems provide a good basis for most simple record-keeping systems for the single or small practice osteopath, although more comprehensive bespoke systems can be purchased. For the osteopath who is to IT what Pavarotti is to bricklaying, it is essential to avoid seeking advice from the gifted amateur. You need a professional. If you want a bespoke system you want a list of criteria that you require to be filled and a clear description of the system to be provided or designed, what it will do, what it will not do and whether and how it would link with other systems, such as those currently in use or under development within the NHS.

As a general piece of advice you should be very careful about rushing into getting a system if the urge takes you. Hospitals and doctors provide a trail of disasters where large sums of money were wasted and huge amounts of time frittered away trying to make an unworkable system work. The best advice is always to use a system that someone else already has working and that you can see demonstrated to your own satisfaction before proceeding to buy one yourself.

In summary, here are the Dos and Don'ts:

- Do make sure that it meets any standards that are required by any relevant authorities and that it is compatible with any other systems with which it may be required to communicate, now *or in the future.*
- Do make sure you know what you want. The all-singing, all-dancing *Pentium 123XYZ* may be brilliant but do you really *need* the specification or will something less spectacular (and cheaper) meet your requirements?
- *Futureproof* your machine. Make sure it does not have obsolescence built into it. It should be upgradeable, flexible and generally OK.
- Don't forget your obligations under the Data Protection Act. If you have any questions, telephone the registrar's office on 01625 545745.
- Think about confidentiality when you have records on the computer. Don't leave screens of information unattended. Don't forget to set up a password, don't use an obvious password like your daughter's first name and don't give your password to anyone else (like the receptionist for instance). However much you trust your receptionist, ask yourself how private detectives find out medical information about patients – it is available if the price is right!
- Back up your files. If you lose data it may be irretrievable and it may cause havoc in your practice. The best advice is:
  - Back up data *every day.*
  - Use new back-up tapes or discs *each day for a week* before considering recycling.
  - Back up critical information *twice a day.*
  - You'll be pleased you took the advice *one day!*
- Don't make it easy for someone to steal your equipment. The local Crime Prevention Officer will be pleased to help.

- Don't get a virus. When you connect up your machine to the big electronic world, the first thing to do is install a reliable virus checker – Norton or Dr Solomon seems to be good.
- Fit a surge protector to your PC's electrical supply. What is it? It is a device for flattening out spikes that occur in the electricity system so that a surge of electricity does not damage the delicate equipment in the PC. A surge can mean blank screens and misery. The device is only a few pounds and well worth the expense.
- Don't allow staff to load games on your PC. They take up disk space and they should not be used; they may introduce nasty viruses into your machine and, anyway, how come they have time to play games?

E-mail is now a ubiquitous communication system. Increasingly it is being used for professional purposes, including referrals, educational exchanges and patient communications. However, with the benefits come some problems and you should be aware of them. The system is simple to use and therein lies one of its major weaknesses. It is easy to pass messages to a large number of people very quickly and those messages can include pictures and graphics. The sign of things to come was heralded by a court case in the United States in 1999 when a large merchant bank agreed a (large) out-of-court settlement with two of its employees because some staff had circulated a joke in bad taste about African-Americans on the internal e-mail. The aggrieved staff reached for their lawyers and the company reached for its chequebook. The court decided that the employers are responsible for internal e-mail traffic regardless of its origin.

☢ Some people try the trick of sticking a blank e-mail in the file every so often so that they can add information at a later stage. It may fool people at a superficial level but don't forget those experts who can work out just what you have done if suspicion is raised.

Since then, legal actions across the world have arisen from allegations about everything from sexual discrimination to breach of confidence in organisations without proper e-mail policies and planning.

If an osteopath were to become involved in a court case or an industrial tribunal, e-mail is ready to provide another shock. A legal device known as **discovery** can be used to force defendants to reveal every file, note and piece of paper they have that might be pertinent to the case in question. Nothing can be hidden. Courts can look in your filing cabinets, your archives and your hard disk too. If they discover that you have deliberately erased e-mails or other electronic documents whilst being investigated you may find yourself in contempt of court. Computer experts can find hidden 'history' and cache files in Windows® and other systems that can leave a trail of clues to what has been done to the files. Emptying the Recycle Bin does not mean gone for good.

If you are using e-mail and particularly if your system has several users, you should consider setting up protocols and guidance fast. Here are the rules:

1 Warn all staff with an on-screen message about the practice's rules for e-mail.
2 Make it clear that e-mail is **not** confidential and will be routinely monitored. Hammer home the fact that e-mail is not a substitute for the kind of conversation that used to take place in the canteen, lavatory or lift.
3 Stamp out any digital gossip. Bar the transmission of personal mail, jokes, smutty material and non-business messages. Experience shows that you may be vulnerable for what any member of your staff does electronically.
4 Set up in-house e-instruction to make sure that staff understand the rules. Incorporate the policies into contracts of employment.
5 Install a programme that monitors e-mail for key words and phrases to flag up offensive material.
6 Decide on archive policies. What will you keep, how long will you keep it and who will be responsible for it?

> Never, never, never, never, never, never, never, never, never, never, never, never open an attachment to an e-mail that has the suffix .EXE unless it came from your mum or the priest. And even then be suspicious. These types of files are a commonly used vehicle for lunatics spreading viruses.
>
> In fact it is wise not to open any e-mail message if you have no idea who the sender is. These days it is possible to screw up your computer with word processing files and all sorts of other material.

REVIEWING THE PRACTICE

How does your place look? The next section is about health and safety but this is about spotting general hazards. The only way to do a proper review is to do a risk management audit. It may sound difficult but it is very easy really. The plan is to find out what can go wrong and to do something about it before it does.

The good news is that this book will help you to sort the thing out with a minimum of aggravation.

SEVEN STEPS FOR IMPLEMENTING A RISK MANAGEMENT SYSTEM

1 *Identify the key risk areas:* The trick here is to involve everyone in the practice. Speak to your staff and ask them where they think the risks are. Have a look at anything that may have gone wrong in the past, check previous insurer contacts if you have had any claims, review any patient complaints and, if possible, talk to patients.

> ✎ If you have 15 minutes and a big enough practice, try the Post-It Note Test. Give everyone some post-its and ask them to make a note and stick it on every dodgy plug, dangly wire, faulty window, etc. It might be a revelation to you.

2 *Identify key trigger events:* Look for trends. History can be a great guide. If it's happened before it may well happen again. Keep an eye open for national incidents – could they happen to you?

3 *Implement an incident reporting system:* Things go wrong everywhere. It is no sin unless you don't do anything about it. Make sure if any staff see a problem they feel comfortable to tell you about it. You need a no-blame

culture. Near misses are particularly important. Furthermore, it is good to learn from our mistakes but a whole lot better to learn from other people's.

4 *Investigate high-risk events:* When something does go wrong, investigate it immediately, even if all the facts are not immediately to hand. Look for the cause and how to avoid a recurrence. If staff are involved, find out their view on what happened but remember that they may be cautious or feel threatened.

5 *Monitor and analyse reports for trends:* You may need an anorak for this. Risk management is about predicting what might go wrong. Be honest and, if necessary, self-critical.

6 *Implement changes in the practice as necessary:* No point in bothering with trends and all that if you are not going to make use of it. If you have staff make sure they all understand why change is necessary. You know what happens if it is done badly – just look at the NHS!

7 *Education and feedback:* Most accidents occur out of ignorance. Make sure everyone knows what has been a problem and why it is no longer a problem now.

You may be able to get further help from:

- the professional indemnity (defence) insurer
- the General Osteopathic Council.

Of course, this book will be the best source!

Finally, if your review throws up a number of problems, use the risk formula to assess the risk:

$$\textbf{Risk} = \begin{array}{c} \text{Likelihood} \\ \text{of} \\ \text{hazard} \end{array} \times \begin{array}{c} \text{Severity} \\ \text{of} \\ \text{consequences} \end{array}$$

Risk factor* = Numerical representation of risk

> * Where 1 is low and 5 is high, allocate a number between one and five to express the likelihood of the hazard and a number between 1 and 5 to measure the potential severity of the consequences. Multiply them together and use that as a numerical expression of relative risk.

What you need is a checklist for your buildings to make sure that there is nothing obvious that may cause you a problem. A building costs a lot of money to build and maintain and it is worth looking after even if only for the sake of making sure it contributes to your pension. More importantly, the public and the staff are in and out of the place, so it must be safe and meet the health and safety standards (more of this in the next chapter).

It is worth walking around the surgery and thinking about it from the perspective of the patients, adults and children, as well as the staff.

Here is a list of the sort of things you should be looking for:

	OK	Not OK	Who will sort it?	By when?

The reception/waiting area
- Is the entrance door easy for a patient to open?
- Is there disabled access?
- Is the reception on one level?
- If doors are fully glazed are there markings to indicate the presence of glass for partially-sighted patients?
- Is glass in doors toughened or laminated?
- Is part of the reception desk at a suitable height for patients in wheelchairs?
- Is there a hearing loop for deaf patients?
- Is there an area where a patient can speak in confidence to a receptionist?
- Is the telephone situated such that patients waiting in reception cannot hear conversations with patients?
- Are there sufficient chairs?
- Are patients kept informed of delays in being seen?
- Are all parts of the waiting room visible to staff?
- Is there adequate heating and ventilation?
- Are carpets free of frays and suitably fitted to avoid the risk of slipping or tripping?
- Are floors safe and not slippery?

Toilets
- Do they meet requirements for disabled access?
- Is there an alarm for a patient unwell or immobile in the toilet?
- Can the toilet door be opened by a staff member from outside?

	OK	Not OK	Who will sort it?	By when?

Consulting room
- Is the room of adequate size, ventilated and heated?
- Is the plinth appropriately located and suitably screened?
- If you use sharps, is the sharps box inaccessible to small children?
- Is the room equipped with a panic alarm?
- Is the floor safe?
- Is the lighting adequate?
- Is the décor of suitable colours for partially sighted patients?

There you are. That should keep you going for a little while but at least the surgery will have no obvious hazards which might end up costing you much more time and heartache.

HEALTH AND SAFETY

Increasingly, practitioners are working in groups and the surgeries from which they practise are becoming their biggest assets. The smart osteopath should be aware of health and safety requirements as they relate to issues ranging from employment to cross-infection.

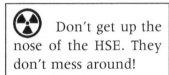 Don't get up the nose of the HSE. They don't mess around!

I suppose that it is just possible that one or two of the readers might not be fully up to date with the health and safety regulations. Well, you should be aware of Section 2 of the *Health and Safety at Work Act 1974*, which details certain responsibilities for all people who work there, whether employed, self-employed or the employer.

Failure to comply can lead to prosecution by the Health and Safety Executive (HSE). The responsible employer (that's you!) must provide and maintain a safe working environment with safe equipment and procedures in place.

It is not all one-way. Employees have responsibilities too. They must have due regard to health and safety procedures and to report anything that could compromise these to the person in charge (that means you as well!).

Health and safety legislation is becoming more risk-led. There is a specific duty to employers to assess the risks to which their employees are exposed. The requirement to assess risks may be general (Management of Health and Safety at Work Regulations 1999) or specific (COSHH Regulations).

Under health and safety law the employer is required to display various things. These are they!

- A health and safety poster, 'Health and Safety Law – what you should know', in the practice to ensure compliance with the Health and Safety Information for Employees Regulations 1989.
- A current certificate of employer's liability.

- A written Health and Safety Policy. This is a requirement of practices with five or more employees and it should be brought to their attention.
  What goes into such a policy?
    - a statement of the employer's commitment to providing a safe and healthy working environment
    - details of safe working practices
    - details of responsibilities for health and safety throughout the workplace.

The HSE is the statutory body responsible for enforcing the Health and Safety at Work Act and its inspectors have the power to inspect premises to ensure that they comply with regulations. They may ask to see the written health and safety policy statement.

If there are concerns about premises the HSE has the power to enter to inspect and if breaches of the legislation are identified, the HSE inspector can issue an improvement notice or a prohibition notice. Prosecution could result in a hefty fine.

Other Health and Safety at Work Regulations came into force on January 1 1993. They implement EC directives and update existing law. They cover:

- general health and safety management
- work equipment safety
- manual handling of loads
- workplace conditions
- personal protective equipment
- display screen equipment.

So, to start, check the following:

- Do the premises comply with applicable local building codes and regulations?
- Do you have adequate public liability insurance to cover your premises?
- Is there a certificate of public liability insurance on display?

DUTIES TO STAFF

These are your duties as an employer. Employers must ensure, as far as is practicable, the safety and welfare at work of all employees. This duty

✍ Although it is not necessary in a small practice to give everyone a copy of this written statement, it may be a jolly good idea.

extends to patients and any other individuals who may be legitimately on the premises.

All systems of work must be safe and without risk to health and this applies to all equipment used within the place of work. Equipment must be regularly maintained, serviced and renewed. Safe systems of work must be in place for all persons. You must:

- provide a written policy statement on health and safety if you employ five or more staff
- provide and maintain safe equipment, appliances and systems of work
- assess all equipment and systems of work for risk
- initiate safe systems of work
- maintain the place of work, including the means of entrance and exit, in a safe condition
- provide a working environment for employees that is safe, without risk to health and with adequate facilities and arrangements for their welfare at work
- provide the necessary instruction, training and supervision to ensure health and safety
- arrange safe disposal of waste
- ensure that dangerous or potentially harmful substances or articles are handled and stored safely.

Osteopaths who employ five or more staff must prepare a written statement of the practice's policy *'with respect to health and safety'* of its employees. This must include details of the organisation and arrangements for carrying out this policy and the immediate action required by staff in respect of any accidents that may occur.

Health and safety statements usually consist of three parts:

- a statement of intent which is a declaration of the employer's commitment to providing a safe and healthy workplace and environment
- details of responsibilities for health and safety throughout the workplace
- details of safe systems of work and safe working practices for all work activities.

The statement should also include the practice's policy on violence, infection control and first aid arrangements.

DUTIES TO STAFF CHECKLIST

There's not a lot of options here. It's just got to be done.

	Done	Doing it	Who by?	When?
• Does the osteopath understand the duties to staff?				
• Does the osteopath undertake a risk assessment of the potential hazards of the practice?				
• Does the osteopath review the materials used in the practice?				
• Is the osteopath satisfied that all systems are safe and without risk to health?				
• Does the osteopath with more than five staff provide a written policy statement on health and safety?				
• Does the osteopath maintain the place of work in a safe condition?				
• Does the osteopath provide the necessary instruction, training and supervision to ensure health and safety?				
• If applicable does the osteopath arrange the safe disposal of waste?				
• Are potentially harmful substances handled and stored safely?				
• Does the osteopath strongly advise all staff to be immunised against diphtheria, tetanus, whooping cough, TB, rubella and hepatitis B?				

PREMISES

So far as is reasonably practicable as regards any place of work under his or her control, the osteopath must ensure that the building is maintained in a safe condition without risks to health. There must be a safe means of entrance and exit for staff and patients.

If the practice occupies a rented building or a health centre under the control of a PCT you must do what is reasonable, but you have a duty to maintain what the lease requires you to do, and you should notify the landlord of anything that should be maintained by him, e.g. loose guttering.

If you have made the necessary notification, ideally in writing (and kept a copy), you would be exonerated if an accident occurred. If you take out a lease, have your lawyer take a good look at it to make sure that your maintenance responsibilities are clearly stated in the lease.

Remember, even if you do not own premises, you will continue to be held responsible for hazards such as slippery floors and unsafe electrical flex.

The Act also states that, as far as reasonably practicable, the employer must provide and maintain a working environment for employees which is without risk to health and with adequate provision for their general welfare. The wording appears to apply to more than just the physical environment of the employee. The osteopath would be well advised to consider whether there is an adequate rest room, refreshment facilities and toilet and washing arrangements, etc. The extent to which this can be done depends on the practice's resources.

Alterations to existing buildings and new premises building should take account of health and safety and security aspects of the practice. There should be wide doorways, grab rails, ramps and as few steps as possible to accommodate the elderly and infirm, children and people in wheelchairs and to meet disabled person legislation (see later).

> Is this section relevant? Probably not but beware if you join a group practice.

The law makes provision for staff representatives and safety committees. If you have staff in a union that you recognise and, if two or more safety representatives ask for a safety committee, the employer must set one up. They acquire all sorts of responsibilities and duties.

PREMISES CHECKLIST

	Yes	No	Fix it	By when?	Who?
• Is the building maintained in a safe condition without a risk to health?					
• Do the premises comply with applicable building codes and regulations?					
• Is there a safe means of entrance and exit for staff?					
• Are there designated and clearly marked fire exits?					
• Does/do the osteopath(s) understand who has responsibility for maintaining the building?					
• Is adequate lighting and ventilation provided in all areas?					
• Is there disabled access to the premises?					
• Are there adequate toilet facilities?					
• Is a non-smoking policy in place and enforced?					
• Are there adequate rest and changing areas for staff?					
• Is adequate, comfortable seating available?					
• Is the reception/waiting area visible to the receptionist?					
• Do reception and examination areas assure patients of privacy during interviews, examinations and treatment?					

DUTIES TO OTHER USERS OF PRACTICE PREMISES

The primary purpose of the Health and Safety at Work Act 1974 is to ensure the safety of employees but it also applies to all persons who enter the premises – all visitors, patients and tradespersons such as postmen, window cleaners, builders, electricians, and even your mother-in-law . . .

> ☢ The Act imposes a duty on the osteopath as 'controller' of the premises to ensure the safety of legitimate visitors.

The law requires the osteopath to conduct practice in such a way as to ensure, as far as reasonably practicable, that all persons not in their employment are not exposed to risks to their health and safety.

The Act links up with the Disability Discrimination Act 1995 (see later) and with another Act called the Occupier's Liability Act of 1957, which is too boring to detail but suffice it to say that you should remove any obvious hazards, particularly to the elderly, infirm and disabled.

The key difference between this duty and the osteopath's duty to his or her own staff is that staff should have a written safety policy and have instruction and supervision on safety matters, and specific arrangements should be made for health, safety and welfare.

EMPLOYER'S LIABILITY

The Employer's Liability (Compulsory Insurance) Act 1969 requires an employer to have adequate insurance and to display a certificate to that effect. New regulations came in during 1999 to supplement the 1969 regulations, which remain in force.

> Responsibilities lie with the practice owner and with the staff. Employers and employees should co-operate to provide a safe place of work. Employees should take reasonable care of the own health and safety.

Employers must have £5 million of cover and they will be required to keep certificates of insurance for **40** years.

Practice premises must also be covered by adequate public liability insurance and a certificate to that effect must be displayed. The Occupier's Liability Acts 1957 and 1984 regulate the duty which an occupier of premises owes to his or her visitors in respect of damages due to the state of the premises or to things which have been done to them or which have not been done to them. Generally this means that premises must have adequate lighting, safe stairways and all that sort of commonsense stuff.

Staff are responsible for:

- health and safety with regard to themselves, their colleagues and their patients
- abiding by health and safety rules of the practice
- reporting anything which could compromise health and safety to the person in charge.

Every employee is under a duty not to interfere intentionally or recklessly with, or misuse anything provided for the purposes of health, safety and welfare. This protects appliances and arrangements to ensure people's safety, such as fire escapes, fire extinguishers and hazard warning notices. This could be extended to include interference with anything provided for welfare purposes, such as cloakroom and refreshment facilities.

ENFORCEMENT

The Acts cover all places of employ-ment and the HSE therefore has the right to inspect osteopath practices. The HSE is divided into areas and each has a team of inspectors.

Inspectors have a warrant of appointment that states their exten-sive powers and the osteopath may ask to see this for identification. Inspectors have the right to enter any premises and enforce the Act. They do not have to seek permission or give notice of entry. They may, however, only enter at a 'reasonable time'.

> Inspectors normally give notice of their visits and ring to make an appointment. Occasion-ally a visit may be reactive to a complaint from an employee or a patient, or they may make an unannounced call simply because it fits conveniently into a sche-dule for other premises.

During a visit, an inspector can interview and take written statements from anyone who may have relevant information, including patients as well as staff. The inspector may want information or to establish the facts about an accident or for evidence for legal proceedings. Any information will normally be treated as confidential. The information, however, may be disclosed subsequently if a prosecution is brought against the employer.

WHAT ARE THE INSPECTORS LOOKING FOR?

- A statement of general policy on health and safety and instructions on safety procedures if the osteopath has more than five staff.
- Compliance with the requirement to carry out a risk assessment under the Management of Health and Safety at Work Regulations 1999.
- Evidence of a good general approach to management of health and safety, specifically:
  - a record of accidents
  - electrical equipment which is in safe working order and properly maintained
  - normal standards of toilet and washing facilities

- hot and cold running water: inspectors may also recommend that wrist-operated taps should be fitted in rooms used for examinations and treatment of patients
- condition of the heating plant, storage of drugs if appropriate, condition of sterilisers if used and standards of heating and lighting.

IMPROVEMENT AND PROHIBITION NOTICES

After completing an inspection, the inspector will usually approach the person in administrative charge of the building about any improvements to safety procedures and standards that may be required. If they are minor the inspector will simply ask for them to be put right. If there is something more serious, the inspector may write formally or issue a written notice requiring things to be remedied. This is called an **improvement notice**. It will specify a time limit of not less than 21 days within which the improvement must be made.

> *The inspector should also advise of the procedure for appeal against the provisions of the notice – very comforting!!*

The inspector must inform staff as well as the practice owner of the service of the notice. A prosecution alleging a specific breach of a statutory provision may also be brought.

If there is a serious risk to health and safety, an inspector may issue a **prohibition notice** forbidding the offending work activity. If the position is very grave the notice will take immediate effect and work must stop at once. Otherwise a deferred prohibition notice may be issued stopping the work after a specified time.

Improvement and prohibition notices are both served on the person carrying out or in control of the work in question, normally on the practice owner.

A person on whom notice is served may appeal to an employment tribunal within 21 days of the notice being served. An improvement notice is suspended pending the outcome but a prohibition notice remains in force until the appeal is determined. When complied with, notices cease.

Don't mess with inspectors! They can:

- issue an improvement notice which specifies the legal requirements being broken, what action is required to put matters right and the period of time allowed
- issue a prohibition notice if there is a risk of serious personal injury

- seize, render harmless or destroy any substance or article considered to be the cause of imminent danger or serious personal injury
- prosecute any person contravening a relevant statutory provision, either instead of or in addition to serving a notice. Conviction can result in a fine of up to £20,000 for some offences.

Failure to comply with a prohibition notice can result in a jury trial and imprisonment for up to two years.

Because the Health and Safety at Work Act is a criminal statute, contravention of its provisions may lead to a fine or imprisonment. Both the employer and the staff may be liable for prosecution. Alongside the criminal prosecution, an employee could sue an employer for damages on the basis of employers' liability law, or simply for negligence. Wow!

Time for a cuppa, I think.

FIRST AID AND COLLAPSE ROUTINE

This may be necessary if you have just read the health and safety information!

Under the Health and Safety (First Aid) Regulations 1981 all employers must make adequate first aid provisions. Ideally a first aid person should be nominated and all employees should know where the first aid box is kept.

All staff members (and the osteopath him or herself) should be trained in cardiopulmonary resuscitation and prepared to deal with any emergency.

Apart from any legislative requirements, failure to be able to manage an emergency (cardiac arrest, diabetic collapse, epileptic fit, etc.) will reflect badly on the osteopath and the practice.

A first aid box should be provided and it should contain:

- a guidance card on resuscitation
- individually wrapped sterile adhesive dressings (various sizes)
- individually wrapped triangular bandages
- medium-sized individually wrapped sterile unmedicated wound dressings (approximately 10 cm × 10 cm)

> First Aid Boxes should *not* contain medication of any kind.

- large sterile individually wrapped unmedicated wound dressings
- other wound dressings
- safety pins
- sterile eye pads and attachments.

FIRE SAFETY

The Fire Precautions (Workplace) Regulations 1997 require the employer to assess what fire precautions are needed by carrying out a fire risk assessment under the Management of Health and Safety at Work Regulations 1999.

Employers are required to ensure that proper consideration has been given to fire prevention. The regulations require an employer to ensure various measures are taken:

> If you have a big practice remember that in buildings with more than 20 employees or more than 10 working on floors other than the ground floor, the owner of the premises is required to obtain a certificate from the local fire authority regulating the means of escape and marking fire exits.

- Emergency routes and exits are kept clear of obstructions.
- They should lead directly to a place of safety.
- They should be clearly indicated.
- Fire detection devices and fire fighting equipment should be in good working order and regularly checked.
- A system should be in place ensuring that, in the event of a fire, the number of people in the practice at that time can be identified.

Premises should be equipped with properly maintained alarms and the employees should be familiar with the means of escape and the routine to be followed in the event of a fire. There should be emergency lighting as necessary. Local fire inspectors will ensure that these requirements are complied with.

Make sure that:

- A fire can be detected in a reasonable time and people warned.
- Automatic fire detection is considered.
- People in the building can get out safely.
- There is adequate fire fighting equipment available.

- A fire extinguisher is provided for each 200 square metres of floor space with a minimum of one per floor.
- All employees know what to do in the event of a fire.
- Fire equipment is regularly checked and maintained.

Emergency routes and exits should:

- be kept free of obstruction at all times
- lead directly to a place of safety
- be appropriately and clearly indicated
- have emergency lighting if required
- open in the direction of escape and in an easy and immediate action.

FIRE CHECKLIST

	Yes	No	Will be sorted	By when?	Who by?
• Is all appropriate fire fighting equipment available?					
• Is fire fighting equipment serviced regularly?					
• Are escape routes and exits clear and appropriately signed?					
• Are extinguishers appropriately signed?					
• Are fire and smoke alarms installed, maintained and tested regularly?					
• Are practice staff trained to respond to fire?					
• Is fire drill practised regularly?					
• Is a fire drill notice displayed in the practice?					
• Do staff have written protocols about fire procedures?					

ELECTRICITY REGULATIONS

This time it is the Electricity at Work Regulations 1989. They are concerned with the safety of both the fixed supply to the premises and any moveable (portable) appliances.

Electrical equipment must be in good working order at all times and all earthed equipment and most leads and plugs connected to equipment should have an occasional combined inspection and test by an appropriately trained person to identify any faults which may not be found by a visual check. The HSE has suggested intervals of up to five years in low-risk environments depending on the type of equipment used.

> If someone receives a shock or worse, compliance with legislation in respect of inspection and testing would be vital to your defence.

There are contract electricians who will provide this type of service. They put little stickers on things to show they've tested them. They'll even remember when they last checked your equipment and come round and do it again – when the time (and the price!) is right.

If it is time for ☕ make sure that the electric kettle is safe!

ELECTRICAL CHECKLIST

	Yes	No	Will be sorted	By when?	By whom?
• Have you got a programme for ensuring electrical equipment is safe at all times?					
• Is electrical equipment installed by appropriate contractors?					
• Is all electrical equipment earthed?					
• Is all electrical equipment provided with fuses of the correct amperage?					
• Is electrical equipment maintained regularly and a record kept?					
• Is electrical wiring checked regularly to inspect for cable or plug damage?					
• Are staff vigilant to the possibility of equipment overheating and aware to whom such problems should be reported?					

COSHH REGULATIONS

Maybe you don't use any hazardous substances – breathe a sigh of relief.

The Control of Substances Hazardous to Health Regulations 1999 (COSHH) set out the legal framework for the management of health risks from exposure to hazardous substances used at work. They aim to prevent occupational ill health by encouraging employers to assess and prevent or control risks from exposure to hazardous substances in a systematic and practical way.

The regulations set out the measures that employers and employees have to take. Failure to comply exposes people to risk and constitutes an offence under the

> ✍ The regulations apply to most hazardous substances except those covered by their own legislation, such as asbestos, lead and materials producing ionising radiations.

HSW Act. Hazardous substances include those labelled as dangerous (toxic, harmful, irritant or corrosive).

Osteopaths may have to be careful about certain cleaning fluids, phenolics, formaldehyde or glutaraldehyde used as chemical disinfectants and clinical waste, either in osteopathy or in related specialities.

All employers should consider how COSHH applies to their employees and working environment. For most osteopaths, compliance should be very straightforward.

This is what you do:

- identify hazardous substances
- assess the risk to health and what precautions are required
- record the precautions in writing
- introduce measures to prevent or control exposure
- ensure that control measures are used
- inform and instruct employees about risks and precautions to be taken.

 Waste disposal basic requirements:
- Have a written practice waste disposal policy.
- Arrange for safe transportation and collection of waste and safe disposal in accordance with legislation.
- If in doubt, regard waste as clinical.

Simple!

WASTE DISPOSAL

Waste disposal depends on what you have to dispose of, which in turn reflects the sort of practice you do. The Environmental Protection Act 1990 places a duty of care to sort waste, store it safely in a suitable container and arrange for its safe disposal. There is a requirement to document disposal routes (Environmental Protection (Duty of Care) Regulations 1991). Depending on the activities conducted in the practice, waste must be segregated into clinical, non-clinical, special waste and sharps.

Non-clinical waste is material such as paper, plastic, etc. Clinical waste is contaminated by blood or other body fluids. If in doubt, classify the waste as clinical and dispose of it accordingly.

Clinical waste must be transported in UN approved rigid containers (Carriage of Dangerous Goods (Classification, Packaging and Labelling) and Use of Transportable Pressure Receptacles Regulations 1996). Sharps must be contained in sealable UN-type approved 'sharps' containers to BS 7320.

Clinical waste and sharps must be collected by authorised persons and documentation of the waste content provided and records of transfer held by both parties. Transfer notes may cover repeated transfers up to one year. You must keep the documentation for two years.

Special waste consists of prescribed medicines and other waste classified as irritant, harmful, toxic, carcinogenic or corrosive. You probably haven't got any. If you have, get a copy of the Special Waste Regulations 1996. Gripping stuff!

WASTE DISPOSAL CHECKLIST

	Yes	No	Will be sorted	By whom?	By when?
• Are you aware of the different types of waste and the requirements for the correct disposal of each?					
• Is practice waste correctly categorised, stored and disposed of?					
• Is clinical waste stored in appropriate containers?					
• Are staff trained in its disposal?					
• Do staff only handle clinical waste when using heavy duty rubber gloves?					
• Are systems in place for the correct transfer of waste?					
• Is waste collected by an authorised person?					
• Has the practice checked the certificate of registration of the waste remover?					
• When clinical waste is removed is a signature obtained by the practice?					
• Are transfer notes kept for two years?					
• Are 'sharps' sealed in UN-type approved containers?					
• Does the practice ever create special waste?					

Boy, do you need this!

COMPUTERS

If technology has reached your practice this could be for you! There are responsibilities in two areas.

1 For regular VDU users there are responsibilities under the Health and Safety (Display Screen Equipment) Regulations 1992, to assess the work-place and to take steps to reduce any identified risks. Employees should be trained to use their workstation correctly in order to avoid health problems. The type of training and the date provided should be recorded.
2 Responsibilities under data protection and other legislation regarding the rights of patients concerning confidentiality and access to clinical records.

We've already looked at data protection – if you don't remember it, it's on page 64 *et seq.*

There's not a lot to say, except: brace yourself for the checklist!

	Yes	No	On someone's to-do list	By whom?	By when?
• Who regularly uses Display Screen Equipment?					
• Do computer users include those people continuously at a screen for longer than one hour at a time, using a PC every day or needing to use a PC to do the job?					
• Have the workstations been assessed?					
• Have the workstations been upgraded or changed to rectify any problems with the workstation set-up identified at risk management?					
• Are free eyesight tests regularly offered to all DSE users?					
• Are employees aware that they should report any discomfort in working with DSE?					
• Are computer users instructed and trained in their use?					
• Are records kept of workstation assessments, eyesight tests and results and are corrective appliances offered and details of information and training provided?					

	Yes	No	On someone's to-do list	By whom?	By when?

- Do images on screen flicker or jump?
- Can the user adjust the brightness and contrast controls on the PC? Is instruction required to enable them to do this?
- Can the user tilt or swivel the screen to avoid glare and allow maintenance of a comfortable posture?
- Is the screen clean and are cleaning materials available?
- Is the keyboard tiltable and separate from the screen (apart from wire connections) allowing the user to adjust the keyboard to suit their needs?
- Does the keyboard have a matt surface to avoid reflective glare?
- Is there sufficient space in front of the keyboard to allow users to rest their wrists whilst keying in or resting?
- Is a wrist rest required and, if so, has it been supplied?
- Is a mouse necessary and has a mouse mat been supplied?
- Is the work area provided adequate to accommodate the range of tasks performed?
- Can unessential items be relocated?
- Is a document holder required and has one been provided?
- Does the work chair allow the user to attain a comfortable posture and is the seat adjustable for height, lumbar support and tilt?
- Does the user require a footrest (do the feet reach the floor when sitting) and if so has one been provided?

Environment
- Do the user's legs fit comfortably under the work surface?
- Does the workstation allow a comfortable posture for the user?
- Is lighting appropriate for the tasks being undertaken?
- Is there glare or reflection from the screen and, if so, have steps been taken to control it using window blinds, lighting adjustment or an antiglare screen?

	Yes	No	On someone's to-do list	By whom?	By when?

- Is noise a problem and, if so, what is proposed for its reduction?
- Are temperature and humidity levels appropriate?

Task design and software
- Is the task designed to ensure variety, allowing the user to take regular breaks to undertake other tasks?
- Can users take breaks from the screen at their own discretion?
- Are users involved in the planning, design and implementation of tasks?
- Does the software used enable users to complete tasks efficiently without presenting unnecessary problems or stress?
- Are users fully trained to operate the software used and have further training requirements been identified?
- Does the software provide on-line help and feedback to the user (e.g. as error messages, etc.)?
- Is there a system of task checking (whereby managers can check the amount of work being generated by employees) and are employees aware of this?

MANUAL HANDLING

It would be jolly embarrassing for an osteopath to fall foul of these regulations, the Manual Handling Operations Regulations 1992. They place responsibilities on both the employer and the employee to ensure that handling is reduced to a minimum and mechanical aids are used wherever possible. Training in handling should be given to all staff and employees must use equipment where it is provided. The employer must assess the risks taking into account the loads involved, the environment in which the handling takes place and the individual capacity for carrying out the task.

It would be the height of embarrassment if you hurt your own back – be careful!

PROTECTIVE CLOTHING

The Personal Protective Equipment at Work Regulations 1992 require an employer to provide protective clothing where it is necessary to ensure safe systems at work. PPE made or sold in the UK must carry the CE marking and necessary information. Surgery clothing must be of a material that can be washed at a temperature of 65°C. Eye and hand protection should be provided and the employer must ensure that it is used by the employee if it is required.

☢ Medical gloves for single use (to BS EN 455) should be worn for relevant clinical procedures. Care should be taken when choosing latex gloves as latex is covered by the COSHH Regulations. So there should be no cutting corners with cheap gloves, no matter how persuasive the rep may be.

Further advice is contained in the Medical Devices Agency's (now the Medicines and Healthcare Regulation Agency, MHRA) publication *Latex Sensitisation in the Health Care Setting (use of latex gloves)* (DB 9601).

REPORTING OF INJURIES, DISEASES AND DANGEROUS OCCURRENCES

Also known as RIDDOR (what a ludicrous acronym), the Reporting of Injuries, Diseases and Dangerous Occurrences Regulations 1995 impose duties on employers to notify the HSE of accidents causing death or major injury in the workplace.

They impose a statutory duty on

☢ All accidents must be recorded in a practice accident book but major accidents must be reported to the HSE immediately by telephone and within 10 days on form F2508.

all employers to keep a record of accidents occurring on their premises and to notify the HSE of certain serious accidents. The employer is responsible for reporting any accident or dangerous occurrence and may be responsible for reporting a case of an occupational disease. It is wise to assume that you should report the latter.

Any notifiable accident must be directly notified to the local office of the HSE by telephone. Keep a written record of the call including the name of the civil servant receiving it and details of the accident, occurrence or disease. A written report should be sent to the HSE within 10 days.

Notifiable dangerous occurrences are also defined in the Regulations and include explosion, electrical short circuit or overload attended by fire or explosion, which resulted in stoppage of the plant for more than 24 hours. Accidents involving explosion of an autoclave could therefore be notifiable.

Employers must make and keep a record of all reported injuries and dangerous occurrences. Under the regulations certain types of diseases must also be reported when a person is carrying out work in an osteopath surgery, such as TB.

 What do you report? Here's a list of basics.

- Record any accidents in the practice accident book.
- If a major accident occurs in the practice the HSE must be notified immediately by telephone and within 10 days on form F2508.
- Dangerous occurrences must be reported, i.e. if something happens which does not result in an injury but could have done so.
- If an accident happens to an employee in your practice and causes that employee to be absent for three days or more, the HSE must be notified.
- If an employee suffers from a reportable work-related disease, the HSE must be informed.

If an accident occurs you must record:

- date and time of the accident
- name and occupation of the injured party
- nature of the injury
- where it occurred
- name and address of witnesses and any other relevant information.

WRITTEN RECORDS OF RIDDOR

A record must be kept of all notifiable accidents and dangerous occurrences, so that the employer can monitor these and identify any preventive action that should be taken. Failure to do so could lead to a fine of up to £5000.

Incidentally . . .

An osteopath need not report an accident to him or herself. See, nobody loves you. Not even the Health and Safety Executive.

Major accidents that need to be reported include:

- fractures of the skull, spine or pelvis
- fracture of any bone in the arm or leg (except in the wrist, hand, ankle or foot)
- amputation of a hand or foot
- dislocation of the shoulder, hip, knee or spine
- loss of sight in an eye
- loss of consciousness through lack of oxygen
- any other injury resulting in a person being admitted to hospital as an inpatient for more than 24 hours, unless detained only for observation.

Notifiable dangerous occurrences include:

- explosion
- electrical short circuit.

SAFETY SIGNS

> **Checklist**
> - All safety signs should carry a pictogram.
> - Fire fighting equipment and unobstructed fire-escape routes must be adequately signposted and contain information on assembly points.
> - A safety sign must be displayed locating the first aid facilities and identifying the designated person.
> - You should have a minimum of the following signs within the practice:
>   - *Fire safety signs:* These must provide safety information on escape routes, emergency exits, location of fire fighting equipment and a means of giving warning in the event of fire.
>   - *First Aid:* Where first aid facilities are located and the designated person.

If you are into details about safety signs, try the Health and Safety Executive. However, here are the basics.

The Health and Safety (Safety Signs and Signals) Regulations 1996 apply to all workplaces and place a duty on employers to use a safety sign wherever a hazard exists that cannot be adequately controlled by any other means.

This means that, when everything else has been done to remove the hazard, safety signs should be used to reduce the risk further. Fire safety signs are within the Regulations and include information on emergency exits, escape routes and the identification of fire fighting equipment.

VENTILATION

The Workplace (Health Safety and Welfare) Regulations 1992 require enclosed workplaces to be ventilated with sufficient fresh or purified air.

This is what the politicians dreamed up – doesn't seem too difficult, does it?

- Windows must be of reasonable size and able to be opened.
- Any air supply must be from a clean source.
- Sufficient air movement must be available.

RADIATION HAZARDS

If you have the facilities to do X-rays then there is another load of regulations with which you must comply. Compliance is required with the Ionising Radiations Regulations 1999, which revoke the 1985 Regulations of the same name. The Ionising Radiation (Medical Exposure) Regulations 2000 revoke the Ionising Radiation (POPUMET) Regulations 1988.

It will come as no surprise that the Ionising Radiation (Medical Exposure) Regulations 2000 place duties on employers and practitioners/operators of radiation equipment.

- The employer shall ensure that written protocols are in place for every type of standard radiological practice for each piece of equipment.

In order to comply with the regulations:

- Notify the local Health and Safety Executive of radiation usage in the practice.
- Decide if a Radiation Protection Adviser (RPA) is required.
- Appoint a Radiation Protection Supervisor (RPS).
- Ensure that equipment meets required standards of radiation safety.

- Provide local rules to all involved, which must include the name of the RPS, a description of the controlled area and any special provisions of a local nature.
- A radiation safety assessment must be carried out every three years by a 'competent authority'. This will be either the National Radiological Protection Board or a local medical physics department.
- All equipment must meet all standards as recommended in 1994 guidelines and must be serviced and maintained according to the manufacturer's specifications.
- Personal monitoring for staff by a dose meter may be required according to the number of X-rays taken per week.
- Staff must be appropriately trained.
- Local rules must include a contingency plan to specify what needs to be done following equipment malfunction.

I expect you really need this now!

HEALTH AND SAFETY (DISABILITY)

If you employ staff you need to read this. On October 1 2004, for the first time, the Disability Discrimination Act will apply to small employers (not those less than 5 feet tall, those with fewer than 15 staff).

☑ Look at the website www.disability.gov.uk.

The topic is worthy of a separate chapter because it will have such a profound effect on all healthcare premises. It is almost certain that your practice does not employ more than 15 staff. If you do, you will know all about these already.

Effectively the Act means that you must be careful not to discriminate against disabled employees or job applicants because of their disability and you may have to consider making reasonable adjustments to your workplace. So, what is a reasonable adjustment? Under the Act you only need to make changes that are reasonable. There are no set rules. Different people, patients and organisations have different needs. Some organisations can afford to do more than others. It is about practicality and availability of resources.

Reasonable changes for employers may include:

- rearranging furniture so that it is not an obstacle course for the disabled
- rearranging duties to accommodate a disabled employee
- allowing someone to work more flexible hours
- allowing someone time off for rehabilitation or treatment
- making arrangements for information handling for a blind person
- providing equipment for a hearing-impaired person.

☢ If someone thinks you have discriminated against someone you can be taken to a tribunal and compensation could be awarded.

✍ If you need information about any aspect of the legislation contact the Department for Work and Pensions on 0845 124 9841 or e-mail DDAinfopack@meads-ltd.co.uk.

Clearly what can be done will depend on the individual circumstances, design of premises and resources available to the osteopath.

The disability legislation does not simply apply to any employees. There is a load of duties already in place for you as a service provider under the Disability Discrimination Act.

You cannot refuse to treat a disabled patient or provide a lower standard of service to a disabled person because of their disability. You should make reasonable changes to the way that you provide your service so that your disabled patients do not suffer discrimination. You should, for example, adjust any natural barriers that may prevent disabled people using your service. The changes that you would need to make are **only those that are reasonable**. It would not be reasonable for an osteopathic practice with (say) one or two osteopaths to make major structural changes to the premises at huge cost. You must consider what is practicable and what resources are available. The law will not require you to make changes that are impractical or beyond your means. You should consider:

- ensuring that the premises are well lit
- ensuring that clear signs are provided
- ensuring the seating is appropriate for disabled patients, i.e. not too low or inaccessible
- using ramps and handrails at the entrance to a building
- ensuring that door handles are of an 'easy-grip' variety
- lowering part or all of the reception desk to make it more accessible for people who use wheelchairs
- using colour contrast to ensure that entrances and exits are easier to use
- seeing disabled patients on the ground floor if your surgery is on two levels.

☑ Don't forget those advice sheets about accessibility. The Disability Rights Commission, which is an independent body, publishes *A Practical Guide for Small Businesses*, which is free. Or visit the DRC website.

Decisions to modify the surgery premises will depend on your individual situation and the disabled patients that you have. It is certainly worthwhile to incorporate disabled-friendly changes in any new building or refurbishments that you might be making. Remember, too, that such modifications will also help the elderly who, though not actually disabled, may appreciate easier access, patients with children, patients with heavy shopping bags or the friends and families of disabled patients.

If you have some disabled patients it might be worth asking their views about the surgery and discussing with them what can be done. Better to work with disabled patients if possible.

UNDERSTANDING DISABILITY: FACT SHEET PUBLISHED BY DISABILITY.GOV.UK

The fact sheet points out that there are 10,000,000 disabled people with wide-ranging impairments covered by the legislation. It is worth reviewing your premises to provide good access and service to patients. The chart below is modified from the leaflet.

Type of impairment	Accessibility issue	Customer service value
Mobility	• Width of doorways and aisles – consider width required for wheelchair access • Height of counters and handles • Evenness of flooring inside and outside the premises • Accessibility of WC facilities	• Ensure suitable seating which is easily accessible • Sit down to talk to wheelchair users so they do not need to crane their neck to see you • Do not lean on the wheelchair. It is part of their personal space
Sight	• Colour contrast on signs, between floors, walls, ceilings and doors • Literature and signage • Clutter and hazards – keep floors clear	• Identify yourself when speaking to a blind person • Stand still so a partially sighted patient can focus on you • If guiding someone, allow them to hold your arm rather than vice versa • Do not move away without telling them
Hearing	• Write down messages if necessary • Add additional aids such as hearing loops • Have visual and audible alarm systems	• Maintain eye contact with lip-reading patients • Speak normally, keep hands away from mouth • Minimise background noise
Speech	• Consider disability awareness training to help staff communicate effectively • Clear signage and labelling	• Speak slowly and clearly • Be patient and listen. Do not speak for the patient • If you do not understand, ask them to repeat themselves • If possible, ask questions with yes or no answers

Type of impairment	Accessibility issue	Customer service value
Learning disabilities	• Signage, clear and concise • Plain English with pictures and images	• Be patient and listen • Ask the person to repeat themselves • Speak clearly and use pictures and symbols

Accessibility to the premises

Checkpoint	Practical suggestions

Approaching and entering

Checkpoint	Practical suggestions
Can disabled people park nearby?	• Disabled parking bays? • Give information or advice about parking
Is the entrance easy to find?	• Make the door a different colour from adjacent windows • Make the name and number clearly visible. Signs perpendicular to the building may be useful
Is the entrance wide enough for all users?	• Consider width for wheelchair users • If doorway cannot be widened, install doorbell • Have glass panels in front door to see who is outside
Is the front door at street level?	• Install permanent or temporary ramp alongside steps • Provide alternative entrance accessible for all users • Speak to local council about street adjustments
Is door easy to open?	• Place door handle at accessible height for wheelchair users • Use easy-grip handle • Install magnetic device that holds doors open • Consider low-energy automatic door opener

Moving around

Checkpoint	Practical suggestions
Is it easy to get round premises?	• Ensure doormats are flush with floor and avoid bristle matting • Remove clutter, eliminate slippery floors • Put handrails on each side of stairs. Consider ramp or lift
Signage	• Keep simple, short and clear • Have good contrast with background, e.g. black on white • Use visual or pictorial symbols in addition to words
Is lighting good?	• Keep windows, lamps and blinds clean • Avoid glare • Light faces from in front rather than behind • Use extra lighting to highlight internal steps and safety hazards
Are floors, walls, ceilings and doors easily distinguishable?	• Use matt paint in contrasting colours or different tones
Is the alarm system and procedure effective?	• Supplement audible alarms with visual alarms • Ensure staff know how to assist disabled people in emergency

Checkpoint	Practical suggestions
Using facilities	
Are your staff skilled in handling disabled patients?	• Allow more time • Talk to the disabled person, not to the companion • Have notepads for exchanging notes • Consider disability awareness training
Can all patients access services?	• General review of access in practice and if possible have a consulting room on the same level as the entrance/waiting area
Seating	• Use flexible seating, of different heights with and without armrests • Have space by chair(s) for a wheelchair to pull up alongside a seated companion
Toilet facilities	• Adequate disabled access to toilet • Wheelchair accessible standards including getting to and from the toilet • Ensure toilet door can be opened with appropriate device from the outside • Provide an alarm pull
Are alternative facilities available if modifications cannot be made?	• Consider providing the service in an alternative location, either by appointment or regularly • Provide an at-home service and ensure that patients are aware of it

It is worth thinking about disabled access **now** if you haven't already done so. Your patients will be pleased you did and you may well help out more people than simply those who have some sort of handicap. It has got to be done, so go and do it.

EMPLOYMENT ISSUES AND RISK

Employment issues are a minefield that is really outside the scope of this book. The legislation regarding the employment of staff is complex and changes more often than David Beckham's hairstyle.

If you are a sole practitioner and are contemplating the employment of staff you should obtain appropriate advice. If you already have staff and you do not feel that you may have done everything by the book or if you feel that a problem might be brewing and you want to be well informed before it does, a good place to start is with the Internet. There are two most helpful sites that can provide you with information about how to deal with employment issues:

- the Advice, Conciliation and Arbitration Service (ACAS): www. acas.org.uk
- the Department of Trade and Industry (DTI): www.dti.gov.uk.

RECRUITMENT AND EMPLOYMENT: SOME BASIC CONSIDERATIONS

Hiring staff of the right quality and skill level is a great talent. You must develop the mentality of a recruiter. It is easy to be impressed by the wrong things. You need to have clear objectives even when recruiting a part-time receptionist. The wrong receptionist can easily cause damage to your reputation, your income and your cardiovascular system if you get cross and frustrated. There are three levels of 'fit' that you may want to consider:

- **Practice fit:** What kind of employee are you seeking? Are you looking for initiative, problem solving, customer care skills or simple administrative function?

- **Team fit:** Would your new employee bring the right qualities and personality?
- **Role fit:** Does your potential new employee have the appropriate technical and other skills and qualifications?

Consider how you are going to find your new employee. It is a dangerous approach to interview someone who is someone's daughter or the next-door neighbour of a friend of yours. You may well end up with a totally inappropriate employee, an acrimonious dismissal and damage to friend or family relationships.

Produce a job description with the required skills and competencies including hours, details of role, required computer and communication skills and any other ancillary competencies such as book keeping, advertising or support for your clinical work. If you expect your new employee to make your tea and buy your Hobnobs, you should tell him or her. The employee should not be surprised by the nature or scope of their role once they have started work. It is also worth making explicit the salary arrangements so that there are no embarrassing discussions about money at a later stage.

Decide where you will place an advertisement. It may be on local notice boards, the local newspaper, using the local employment service or through other routes. By all means include in your interviews those people who are recommended for the role by friends or relatives but explain at the outset that you will review them using the same criteria as for other interviewees. Think **very carefully** before you consider a patient for a staff role.

Once you have received your applications it will be necessary to plan your interviews. Read all the applications carefully. Look out for unexplained gaps in the previous employment history and beware of those *curricula vitae* that are too good to be true; they usually are! Score the applications against the skills and competencies that you seek.

Do not allow racial or other bias to creep into your assessment.

Take up references of potential employees if they have agreed that you may do so before interview. Many likely employees will not want you to tell their existing employer that they are looking for a new job and so will only permit the taking of a reference once you have offered the post.

Plan your interview. You may want to arrange a pre-interview if you have had a number of candidates who appear to meet your requirements and where you need to do some list pruning before the formal interview occurs. The pre-interview will probably be better done out of surgery hours so that you can take the opportunity to show the candidate the practice and explain the details of any tasks that might be unfamiliar (for example operating an autoclave). It also gives the opportunity for the candidate to decide whether the job is really the sort of post for which he or she is looking. Better to have an applicant withdraw at that stage than two weeks after starting the job. You should aim to reduce the number of candidates for a single post to no more than three.

There is little worse than a candidate confronted by an interview panel that hasn't planned its questions in advance. You should consider carefully who will actually do the interview. Should you do it alone or should you create a small panel? The bigger the panel, the more complicated and sometimes clumsy the process is, but to have one or two other people who can offer independent views may be very valuable in helping you to make your decision. Remember that a panel of seven to interview someone applying for a 10-hour-a-week receptionist post would be huge overkill.

Share the questions out between panel members and make sure that you ask all the key questions to which you wish to know answers. Always check what their resignation arrangements are if they are in current employment and the date on which they can start if offered the post.

Once you have made your decision, make clear that any job offer is subject to satisfactory references and **always take up the references** if you have not already done so. Discovering that your new employee has been convicted of a variety of criminal assaults two weeks after being in post is bad news!

Once you have done the checking and are satisfied that the candidate is the employee for you, telephone him or her to make a firm offer. It is friendly and welcoming. Confirm the offer in writing, incorporating confirmation of the principal elements of the post including hours and salary.

Once the new employee is in post you need to ensure that he or she has:

☑ If this is your first employee make sure you do things right and make proper arrangements for payment. Paying cash out of the petty cash should not be the method of choice unless clearly sanctioned by your accountant. He or she will help you to get the payment arrangements properly sorted.

- a job description (best practice)
- a contract of employment providing the terms and conditions of that employment.

The contract should normally have the following components within it:

- title of post
- key elements of role
- hours and place of employment
- holiday entitlement, types of leave and accumulation of leave
- probation period (if applicable)
- remuneration and overtime payments
- payment of bonuses (if applicable)
- illness and certification
- disciplinary procedure
- grievance procedure
- counselling
- unilateral changes.

The employee should be provided with a written statement of the terms and conditions within 13 weeks of the commencement of the employment.

Many of the problems that arise during the course of employing staff relate to failures of communication. Much of this can be eliminated by having a handbook that informs the staff member of the elements of the employment in more detail. It may also contain policies referred to in the contract. Although it may seem to be 'over the top' to give a receptionist an employee's handbook when there may only be one or two staff members, it does provide a way of ensuring that ambiguities within the professional relationship are minimised.

The handbook may contain the following elements.

A STATEMENT OF YOUR EXPECTATIONS OF THE STAFF MEMBER

You can use this section to describe the way in which you would expect a staff member to work and behave and to manage patients. You might want to comment on the issues surrounding the acceptance of patients, any expectations you might have in terms of collecting information about them and what to do if a patient is difficult or behaves inappropriately. You might also want to take the opportunity to include a list of generic tasks or to make reference to the job description.

APPRAISAL

You should have an annual appraisal system for your staff member. There may be circumstances where either you have a problem with them or they have a problem with you or the role within the practice. Providing an opportunity to review the year, to assess the progress of the practice, to identify any difficulties in its operation, to review the employee's role and to consider educational needs and opportunities for development is often very valuable and will allow you to make your business more successful.

ABSENCE

In small businesses the absence of a staff member may have a very serious effect on the function of the practice. You may wish to try to minimise the disruption by asking the staff member:

- to let you know by (say) 9.00 a.m. if he or she is sick and cannot work
- to provide a self-certificate for the first seven days of illness
- to provide a medical certificate for longer periods of illness
- to ensure that he or she is fit to return to work before doing so
- to co-operate if you wish to make enquiries from his or her medical advisers to understand the absence from work.

MATERNITY LEAVE

You may wish to record details of taking time for antenatal appointments, the employee's rights in respect of returning to work after a pregnancy, payments made during maternity leave and any other information you may wish to give.

HOLIDAY ENTITLEMENTS

The number of days off per year, arrangements for public holidays, etc.

DISCIPLINARY PROCEDURES

This is a difficult area but, if problems arise with a staff member and there is no documented disciplinary or grievance procedure, it will be far more difficult to take effective action to control the situation. The procedure must be fair and equitable. It is certainly not beyond the bounds of possibility that you might employ a receptionist about whom, for example, you receive repeated complaints about attitude. Action will be necessary and, if you get it wrong, you may encounter difficulties, particularly if you feel that she should be dismissed.

Disciplinary action should occur only infrequently and the procedure is designed to ensure that there is fair and prompt action. The aim is to bring about improvement through guidance, training and encouragement.

The disciplinary procedure consists of four stages:

1 verbal warning
2 first written warning
3 final written warning
4 dismissal.

The level at which the procedure starts depends on the seriousness of the offence.

You may wish to describe how you will administer the disciplinary process at any given stage.

Employees have a right to appeal against any disciplinary action taken against them.

The disciplinary policy notified in the contract may be included in the handbook.

GRIEVANCE

You will want to create an environment where, if the employee has a problem with his or her employment, he or she feels able to raise it with you, so that you can attempt to deal with it quickly and satisfactorily.

The grievance policy notified in the contract may be included in the handbook.

COMPUTER AND VISUAL DISPLAY UNIT (VDU) USAGE

See the section on IT to notify the employee of the conditions of use of computers (*see* pages 93–6).

ELECTRONIC MAIL

The purpose of the e-mail is to conduct professional business.

Messages and e-mail equipment are the property of the practice.

You reserve the right to access and disclose the contents of all messages created, sent or received using your e-mail system.

E-mails should be treated in the same way as all other professional communications.

E-mails should not contain material that may be considered offensive or disruptive. Offensive content includes but is not confined to obscene or harassing language or images, racial, ethnic, sexual or gender specific comments or images that would offend someone on the basis of their religious or political beliefs, sexual orientation, national origin or age.

Occasional personal use of the e-mail system is permitted, but such messages become the property of the osteopath and are subject to the same conditions as other e-mail.

Violation of the policy will result in disciplinary action up to and including termination of employment and/or legal action if warranted.

HEALTH AND SAFETY

It is necessary to lay out the principles of health and safety. A staff member must ensure that his or her health and safety and that of other users of the practice are not affected by any activity that he or she does or does not do at work.

Your staff should minimise the possibility of an accident. If the staff member identifies a hazardous process it should immediately be brought to your attention.

All accidents at work should immediately be reported to you. Circumstances that might result in injury or damage must also be reported.

Staff must comply with any local safety rules.

The issues to be listed can be found in the chapter 'Health and safety' (*see* page 101) and include:

- Fire safety:
  - fire drill
  - fire alarm
  - fire extinguishers.
- First aid equipment.
- Storage of materials:
  - filing cabinets
  - storage cupboards.
- Lifting: Before you lift, ensure that the area is clean and tidy. Remove any obstacles from the area that may cause a fall, slip or trip, such as trailing

wires and cables, loose carpeting or items of office furniture, and get close to the load.

Assess the weight to be lifted before attempting to do so.

The practice of lifting and handling is based on the following six principles:

- **feet:** hip-width apart with one foot forward in the direction of travel
- **knees:** bend to gain lifting power from the leg muscles
- **back:** straight but not necessarily vertical, to ensure that the spine and the back muscles do not take the strain of the lift
- **hands:** grasp object to be lifted by using the whole of the fingers and the palms of the hands
- **arms:** keep them as close to the body as possible, with elbows well tucked in
- **head:** chin tucked in with head facing the direction in which you intend to move.

Key points:

- Think before lifting.
- Use mechanical aids, e.g. trolley.
- Push, don't pull.
- Obtain assistance for heavy or awkward loads.
- Wear sensible footwear.
- Avoid wearing loose clothes.
- Load at waist height.
- Make sure that you can see over the load.
- Electrical equipment: dos and don'ts.
- Accidents: what to report and to whom.
- COSHH: As applicable to the practice.

ISLAM IN THE WORKPLACE

Muslims now form the largest religious group in the UK. At a time when considerable misunderstandings and stereotypes circulate in the media and society with respect to the religion, it is crucial to make the effort to go beyond stereotypical images and to understand Islam and the Muslim faith. The population contains approximately 1.5 million Muslims and you may well employ staff with the Muslim faith. With a little planning, any sensitivity can be accommodated easily and work relationships can be most satisfactory. In order to retain Muslim employees, you may consider the following:

- prayer periods
- attendance at the mosque
- fasting periods
- dress codes
- religious holidays
- food requirements and restrictions
- physical contact.

If Muslim employees do not feel comfortable it is likely that they will seek employment elsewhere and you may lose an excellent part of the practice team.

Remember that employment rules and regulations are complicated. Seek advice before making precipitate changes in employment arrangements. A well-motivated and committed staff will be worth its weight in gold to you and the smooth running of your practice. It is well worth investing some effort in getting it right.

RISK AND THE MEDIA

There are more and more stories in the newspapers and on radio and television about health. Some are good and some are, well, not so good. A generation ago, medical stories were rare

☑ If you are ever asked for an interview of any sort, always get advice from the insurer's medico-legal adviser.

and virtually only about good news, lives saved, new medical developments, etc. Nowadays many of the items report healthcare professionals who are dishonest, incompetent or frankly whacky! The image of all aspects of healthcare is damaged by these continuous assaults.

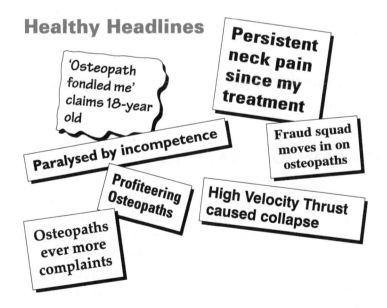

Healthy Headlines

'Osteopath fondled me' claims 18-year old

Persistent neck pain since my treatment

Paralysed by incompetence

Fraud squad moves in on osteopaths

Profiteering Osteopaths

High Velocity Thrust caused collapse

Osteopaths ever more complaints

Increasingly journalists are seeking opinions and interviews from more and more healthcare professionals, including osteopaths. If you are approached there may be two possible reasons why your views are being sought:

- You may find yourself asked to contribute to an item on a particular treatment, maybe because you are known to favour its use, or because you live in close proximity to someone else or a group of other osteopaths who have different or varied views.
- You may be contacted as an expert witness, by virtue of previous broadcasting, public speaking, learned articles or reputation to comment on a particular treatment or approach to illness or disease.

There is, of course, a third reason why you might be contacted for a comment or a statement – because you are at the centre of a storm about your treatment or care of a patient or there are allegations of professional misconduct.

In the latter case **it is vital that you contact your insurer immediately and seek the advice of the in-house medico-legal advisers.** You may need a lot of help to keep you out of difficulties. Fortunately, difficulties of this sort are relatively rare but anyone can suffer an unpleasant or unsavoury allegation and if badly handled the damage to personal reputation, professional standing or family can be considerable.

This section is designed to give pre-warning so that, if you are accosted by a journalist or asked to do a television or radio interview, you know a little of what is expected. The odds are against it but, like the boy scouts, it is best to be prepared.

Many of the principles of dealing with journalists are common to all media but there are particular features associated with each form and it is worth bearing them in mind.

NEWSPAPER JOURNALISTS

This situation is not unknown and people find themselves accosted by a journalist in the hope that, in the heat of the moment, they will say something that gives him a story. You see it all the time, both in the papers and on television, and it is frequently the case that, when pressed to make comments, they are not the best or most appropriate.

If you are confronted by a journalist in this or any similar way, **do not agree to make any comments.** However, if you refuse to speak to them, you expose yourself to the risk that the refusal will be translated into obstruction or carry the implication that you have a guilty secret to conceal. Many people think that the best approach is to decline to comment at that time (giving a reason such as the fact that you have patients to see) but offering to meet the journalist at a mutually convenient time (say) later in the day. This will often be good enough and will satisfy the journalist. It will give you the time to contact the insurer for advice and to prepare yourself to speak to him.

> ☺   You have become concerned about the way in which a local GP is treating back pain sufferers. You have advised your patients not to consult the GP and somehow this information has attracted the notice of the local newspaper. One day you arrive at the practice and, as you walk to the door, a journalist appears and starts questioning you about your reasons for believing that your treatment is better or more appropriate than that of your professional colleague.
>
> What do you do?

Journalists have a job to do like everyone else. Their manner may be inquisitive, probing, intrusive or downright aggressive, but they will be diligent because they need the story. So, how should they be handled?

1 **Contact your insurer:** Discuss with the medico-legal adviser how the situation should be handled. It may be that you can handle the interview yourself, depending on the content and nature of the matter being discussed, or it may be that you need some help from the adviser who may, if necessary, be there with you.
2 **Be prepared:** Collect your thoughts about the issue and make sure that your knowledge is sufficient. Look up any information about which you are not sure in advance so that you can answer any professional questions authoritatively.
3 **Prepare a written statement covering the issues to be discussed:** Give the journalist a copy of the statement. The likelihood is that he will use it as the basis for his article.
4 **Stick to the facts:** Don't allow yourself to be drawn into speculation. Never comment on events outside your area of expertise.
5 **Be positive.**
6 **Bear in mind that you need a patient's consent** before you comment about anything that a patient may have said. In general, it is wise not to comment in any way about a patient. There are exceptions, particularly if you are acting as a patient's advocate (for example to get improved services) but in such a case it is sensible to have the patient's written

consent. Do not be drawn into criticising the patient or making reference to his or her clinical or personal information in response to remarks attributed to the patient about you.

7 **Beware the 'golden question':** Some journalists will have a pleasant, non-aggressive and amiable interview and then make an aggressive or insulting comment, catching the interviewee by surprise. They then ask the one question to which they really want the answer (do you really earn £200k a year, did you sleep with the patient, etc.) in the hope that you may be unsettled by the previous remark and they can catch you off-guard so that you answer, well, more honestly than you might have done. **Do not respond to insults.**

Make sure that you see everything that is written in the paper or magazine about you and keep in touch with your insurer so that any concerns can be handled effectively.

TELEVISION JOURNALISM

It is again the case that there may be a number of reasons why you are required for a television interview:

- You are an expert.
- You are commenting on a case involving another osteopath.
- You are the 'star' of an investigative programme such as *Watchdog*.
- You are explaining an osteopathic technique on a purely factual basis.

It is clear that different strategies are required for different types of interview request, if you agree to do one. If the interview is in any way contentious you should **contact your insurer** immediately and seek advice. I shall confine the advice in this section to the simpler and less inquisitional types of interview.

The television journalist's watchword is preparation. It will usually have been done by a researcher and generally they are very good. You may indeed be surprised by how much they appear to know about your subject. You must remember this if you agree to appear in an interview.

If you do agree to appear, you will be excited at the prospect, you will be nervous and you will be inquisitive to see how everything works. However, when you arrive at the studio, you will probably be gripped by fear, especially if it is your first exposure to the media, and you will probably wish that you hadn't agreed to participate.

Remember the **top ten television tips** for handling an interview of this sort:

1 **Don't do it** unless you feel sure that you are able to. However flattered you may be to have been asked, think carefully. You must **never** assume that, because you are an osteopath, you will either know the answers or be able to bluff it. If you aren't an expert, don't expose yourself. Remember the old saying: *'They may think you are an idiot. Don't open your mouth and prove it!'*

2 **Dress appropriately:** Do not look as though you have just finished the gardening. You need credibility with your audience and therefore you need to dress in a way that is consistent with your professional status. It will be much more difficult for you if you have to overcome a 'credibility gap'. Consider the following:

   (a) **Suit:** To look professional you might consider this appropriate. If so, ensure that the button is done up to look formal.

   (b) **Do not wear your Hawaiian shirt:** A simple, plain, light-coloured shirt is best.

   (c) **Tie:** Do not wear a tie with tight circles or heavy patterns on it. On camera, an interference pattern makes the circles look as though they are spinning like Catherine wheels (a phenomenon called 'strobing'). This distracts from what you are saying.

   (d) **Thin blouses:** Women should be careful not to wear blouses that are very lightweight because the bright television lights may pick out the bra underneath and it can be distracting.

   Overall, the message is to be *quietly professional* and provide the appearance that your audience would expect to see.

3 **Don't drink beforehand:** You do not need a drink beforehand as a loosener. Sometimes, particularly with some of the public debating programmes, speakers are taken to a hospitality suite first. If they have a few drinks they are much more likely to make comments that are 'newsworthy'. Have soft drinks only if you are invited to hospitality.

4 **Demeanour and presentation:** Your general appearance is important. If you look like Shrek it is hard to make you look like Jude Law or Jennifer Aniston. However, there are a number of things you can do to look your best.

(a) Find out whether you will be sitting or standing for the interview. This is important because you will need to consider different issues in terms of appearance.

(b) Go to the loo. Don't wish you had gone halfway through the interview.

(c) Look in a mirror. Make sure your hair looks right and that your tie is straight.

(d) If you are sitting:
  (i) Sit up straight.
  (ii) As you sit down, hold the sides of your jacket at the lower edge and pull it down as you sit down. If you do not do so, you may end up with the jacket sticking up with the collar in a V-shape behind you. It does not look cool.

(e) If you are standing, *don't slouch*.

(f) Remember that studio lights are bright. If they are shining in your eyes you may find yourself squinting during the interview. Mention it. A technician will adjust them.

(g) If you wear variable tint lenses, remember that under studio lights they will become dark. Don't wear them unless you absolutely have to in order to avoid looking as though you are a member of the mafia.

(h) If you are nervous and your hands are shaking, keep them out of the way. Hold the side of your chair. Don't wave them about.

(i) Don't fidget, and . . .

(j) Don't forget to **smile**. A constant serious expression can generate feelings of doubt. However, **caution**: do not be seen smiling at an inappropriate point in an interview. Smile only with good news, not with bad news.

5 **Understand the set-up of the interview in advance.** The most important (and obvious) thing to know is whether it will be live or recorded.

(a) If it is recorded, you can stop an answer if it is going wrong. Discuss it with the interviewer before you start. He or she will not mind you re-recording an answer. Indeed, they may wish to re-ask the question. Some people suggest that you should spoil a wrong answer with rude words or a silly face so that they are not used. In general there is no need to do so. You can ask the studio to see the recording but they may not be able to let you or have the time to do so.

(b) If the interview is live, more care is needed. If you embark on an answer and you realise that it is going wrong, try to finish it as quickly as possible. Don't dig yourself a bigger hole!

6 **Don't be a smart-Alec.** Being too clever is *very* dangerous unless you are very good at it. Don't try to outsmart the interviewer. They virtually always get the last word. They will have dealt with clever Dicks before. Avoid jokes. It is easy to offend and irritate and they hardly ever amuse.

7 **When answering, look straight and unswervingly, either at the interviewer or at the camera.** The interviewer will tell you which is preferred. If you look down or away from the camera you are likely to imply that you are being economical with the truth. Looking straight ahead looks sincere. As someone very famous once (nearly) said, 'you will know you're successful when you can fake sincerity'. Looking straight ahead helps with that. Just watch politicians!

8 **When answering questions, watch out for bear traps:**
   (a) Stick to what you know.
   (b) Do not be drawn into areas where you have no expertise.
   (c) Keep the answers specific and to the point.
   (d) If you don't know, *don't guess.*
   (e) Don't get into a dispute with the interviewer.
   (f) Don't react to insults.

9 **Don't walk out.** If the interview gets tough or aggressive, or if you are struggling to answer the questions, you might want to walk out. Do not do so. It does not look good. It suggests you are running away from the questioner and you leave the questioner to make any comments about you that he or she chooses. Interviews are usually quite short. Stick it out.

10 **When all else fails, you may have to take steps to protect yourself from a question that may cause you problems.** It may be that the interviewer has asked you a question to which you do not know the answer but saying that you do not know does not seem appropriate. Alternatively, you may know the answer all too well but don't want to give it. In such cases, there are a number of things you can do:
   (a) Ask the interviewer to repeat the question. It gives you time to think out the answer and, in any case, the interviewer will probably ask the question differently and the second attempt may be easier to answer.
   (b) Look blank and ask the interviewer to rephrase the question. He or she will have to use different words then!
   (c) 'This is an interesting question and some background to the answer may be helpful . . .' allows you to talk about a related subject where you may be able to speak with more confidence without actually addressing the original question.

(d) 'I think that the question you are really asking me . . .' enables you to re-write your own question. Interviewers are (generally) too polite to tell you that you haven't answered their question.

(e) More blatantly you can actually politely correct the interviewer by saying, 'I think a better question would be . . .'. This needs quite a lot of skill because the interviewer will spot this as a manoeuvre and may try to bring you back to the original question.

(f) Finally, you can just ignore the question you have been asked and wander off on an answer to a vaguely related question. If you do so positively, the interviewer may genuinely believe that you believed that to be the question and will be too polite to interrupt.

Good luck!

RADIO JOURNALISM

Radio journalism has a lot in common with television journalism but there are a number of very important differences.

1 You cannot be seen and so you can dress comfortably. There is no need to wear a jacket or tie. Nobody will know.

2 It is commonly the case that, if you are being interviewed, you will not be in the same studio as the interviewer, so you will not have to contend with being watched. It is sometimes the case that, when several people are being interviewed at the same time, none of them are in the same studio. The national radio stations have access to many studios in such diverse places as municipal offices and other public buildings. With local radio stations you are more likely to be asked to go to the radio station itself.

3 As with newspaper journalists, radio journalists may have a particular question or topic where they are seeking an answer. They may be determined in respect of this particular issue and you may find that they doggedly persist with the one question, which they may ask in different ways.

4 Your secret weapon on the radio is silence. **Silence is golden.** If you are asked a question and you are struggling to answer it, say nothing. Radio cannot cope with silences and so the interviewer will have to cut in straight away and fill the gap, either by asking the question again (it will invariably be a bit different and possibly easier) or, if you are in a different studio, by asking whether you are still on the line. Either way it is a reprieve.

Finally, remember that you can only do your best. However good you are, you may be caught out. However careful you are with your answers, an edited answer may sound quite different. After you have done your interview, go home, watch it, listen to it or read it, and enjoy it. Then pour yourself a scotch and forget it. It's over.

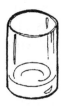

Conclusion

Well, there we are.

I hope that the book has given you some thoughts to ponder about the hazards that face you in general osteopathic practice. You may, of course, be tempted to ask yourself, or me, why the devil you should bother; it will cost you effort, thought and possibly money in some cases to reduce your risk and to make your practice safer. If you don't do anything you may be more vulnerable to an accident or a claim but, hey, that's why you are insured.

Perhaps you should consider that logic a little more carefully. There are several reasons why it is anything but logical to rely on insurance to bail you out.

1 If an accident occurs, you may end up with a patient or even a member of staff (or heaven forbid, you) injured. Your duty to those you treat and who work with you should encourage you to minimise that as a possibility.

2 If you are accused of negligence you may be amazed to discover how popular you are, particularly with the local press. The neighbourhood reporter will be thoroughly fed up with reporting weddings and complaints about dogs fouling the pavement. A juicy story about your negligence, especially if it is a bit lascivious, will go down a storm with the *Middle Wackett Advertiser*. They will run it week after week. Believe me; a bit of risk management is well worthwhile.

3 Negligence may mean a visit to the local, or High Court or to GOsC. Not something that you will want to do.

4 Negligence equals claims. The greater the number of claims, the higher the cost of insurance. You know how you hate having to pay increasing premiums. In the end, the level at which those premiums are set is in your hands. Furthermore, most insurers may think twice about insuring you if they suspect that you are profligate.

5 Perhaps the best reason is that you will probably take a pride in what you do. There is a real buzz when the patient thanks you profusely for curing him or her. You really can't enjoy the patients when things go wrong. Reduce the risk. Bask in the success. Sleep at night!

If you want to be the greatest osteopath in the world, it is almost certain that you won't be able to achieve that without reading this book.

Improving practice, keeping claims down and improving your standard of living – why not? Here's to more power to your elbow.

Good luck!

And *cheers*!

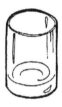

APPENDIX 1: ANSWERS TO EXERCISES

PAGE 56

EXERCISE 1

Consent may be implied, verbal or written. If the patient turns her knee towards you, it is an invitation to look only. Clearly any examination will involve touching the knee and leg and, as such, the normal consent policy must be adopted. Implied consent will not be sufficient.

EXERCISE 2

If you are asked to undertake a treatment about which you are not confident or which you do not believe is appropriate in the particular patient's circumstances, you should not use it because the patient has a belief in it.

You should explain why you propose the treatment plan that you are suggesting and not be drawn into a technique that you do not consider suitable.

If you use the patient's 'cure' and it produces an adverse outcome, you will have to justify its use and suggesting it was because you were asked to use it may not be sufficient.

EXERCISE 3

No.

'Do whatever you need' is not consent. To be able to consent the patient must understand the benefits, disadvantages and consequences of not having treatment.

EXERCISE 4

The osteopath must act in the patient's best interests. It is important to establish that the patient is not competent and does not show periods of competency that might allow her to make a decision. The views of the carers, friends and relatives should be taken into consideration and the treatment considered should be the minimum necessary to assist the patient. Having done so, the osteopath may proceed, but should be careful to write comprehensive notes in case he or she is asked to justify the decision at a later stage.

EXERCISE 5

Yes.

Patients can withdraw consent at any time and you must respect their decision. You can, of course, continue to explain why you need to do what you consider necessary.

PAGE 59

EXERCISE 6

Under normal circumstances the answers are:

- No.
- No.
- No.

APPENDIX 2: THE OSTEOPATHS ACT 1993

All osteopaths work within the framework of the Osteopaths Act 1993. It is probably as well if you actually have a copy just in case you ever need to refer to it.

The Osteopaths Act 1993

ARRANGEMENT OF SECTIONS

An Act to establish a body to be known as the General Osteopathic Council; to provide for the regulation of the profession of osteopathy, including making provision as to the registration of osteopaths and as to their professional education and conduct; to make provision in connection with the development and promotion of the profession; and for connected purposes.

[1st July 1993]

Be it enacted by the Queen's most Excellent Majesty, by and with the advice and consent of the Lords Spiritual and Temporal, and Commons, in this present Parliament assembled, and by the authority of the same, as follows: –

The General Council and its committees

The General Osteopathic Council and its committees.
1. – (1) There shall be a body corporate to be known as the General Osteopathic Council (referred to in this Act as "the General Council").

(2) It shall be the duty of the General Council to develop, promote and regulate the profession of osteopathy.

(3) The General Council shall have such other functions as are conferred on it by this Act.

(4) Part I of the Schedule shall have effect with respect to the constitution of the General Council.

(5) There shall be four committees of the General Council, to be known as –

(a) the Education Committee;

(b) the Investigating Committee;

(c) the Professional Conduct Committee; and

(d) the Health Committee.

(6) The four committees are referred to in this Act as "the statutory committees".

(7) Each of the statutory committees shall have the functions conferred on it by or under this Act.

(8) The General Council may establish such other committees as it considers appropriate in connection with the discharge of its functions.

(9) Part II of the Schedule shall have effect with respect to the statutory committees.

(10) At the request of the General Council, Her Majesty may by Order in Council make such provision with respect to the matters dealt with by the Schedule as Her Majesty considers appropriate in consultation with the General Council.

(11) Any such Order in Council shall be subject to annulment in pursuance of a resolution of either House of Parliament.

(12) Any provision under subsection (10) may be made either in substitution for, or as an addition to, that made by any provision of the Schedule.

Registration of osteopaths

The Registrar of Osteopaths.

2. – (1) The General Council shall appoint a person to be the registrar for the purposes of this Act.

(2) The person appointed shall be known as the Registrar of Osteopaths (referred to in this Act as "the Registrar") and shall hold office for such period and on such terms as the General Council may determine.

(3) It shall be the duty of the Registrar to establish and maintain a register of osteopaths in accordance with the provisions of this Act.

(4) The Registrar shall have such other functions as the General Council may direct.

(5) Where the terms on which the Registrar holds office include provision for the payment to him of any allowances or expenses, the rate at which those allowances or expenses are paid shall be determined by the General Council.

(6) The terms on which the Registrar holds office may, in addition to providing for his remuneration, include provision for the payment of such pensions, allowances or gratuities to or in respect of him, or such contributions or payments towards provision for such pensions, allowances or gratuities, as may be determined by the General Council.

Full registration.

3. – (1) Subject to the provisions of this Act, any person who satisfies the conditions mentioned in subsection (2) shall be entitled to be registered as a fully registered osteopath.

(2) The conditions are that the application is made in the prescribed form and manner and that the applicant –

    (a) has paid the prescribed fee;

    (b) satisfies the Registrar that he is of good character;

Appendix 2: The Osteopaths Act 1993

(c) satisfies the Registrar that he is in good health, both physically and mentally; and

(d) has a recognised qualification.

(3) Where an application for registration is made during the transitional period by a person who was in practice as an osteopath at any time before the opening of the register, he shall be treated as having a recognised qualification if he satisfies the Registrar that for a period of at least five years (which need not be continuous) he has spent a substantial part of his working time in the lawful, safe and competent practice of osteopathy.

(4) For the purposes of subsection (3), no account shall be taken of any work done by the applicant before the beginning of the period of seven years ending with the opening of the register.

(5) For the purposes of subsection (3), the question whether the applicant has spent any part of his working time in the lawful, safe and competent practice of osteopathy shall be determined in accordance with such rules (if any) as may be made by the General Council.

(6) The General Council may by rules provide for treating a person who –

(a) has obtained a qualification in osteopathy outside the United Kingdom,

(b) does not hold a recognised qualification, but

(c) satisfies the Registrar that he has reached the required standard of proficiency,

as holding a recognised qualification for the purposes of this Act.

(7) In this section "transitional period" means the period of two years beginning with the opening of the register.

Conditional registration.

4. – (1) Subject to the provisions of this Act, any person who satisfies the conditions mentioned in subsection (2) shall be entitled to be registered as a conditionally registered osteopath.

(2) The conditions are that the application is made in the prescribed form and manner during the transitional period and that the applicant –

(a) has paid the prescribed fee;

(b) satisfies the Registrar that he is of good character;

(c) satisfies the Registrar that he is in good health, both physically and mentally;

(d) satisfies the Registrar that for a period of at least four years (which need not be continuous) he has spent a substantial part of his working time in the lawful, safe and competent practice of osteopathy;

(e) if required to do so by the Registrar in accordance with rules made by the General Council, passes –

(i) the prescribed test of competence; or

(ii) such part of that test as the Registrar may specify; and

(f) gives the required undertaking.

(3) In the application of subsection (2)(d), in relation to any person, no account shall be taken of any work done by him before the beginning of the period of six years ending with the opening of the register.

(4) The General Council may by rules provide for the conversion, in prescribed circumstances and subject to the osteopath concerned complying with such conditions (if any) as may be prescribed, of conditional registration into full registration.

(5) Unless it is converted into full registration in accordance with the rules, any conditional registration shall cease to have effect –

(a) at the end of the period of five years beginning with the opening of the register; or

(b) where a shorter period has been specified by the Registrar in accordance with subsection (10) in relation to the osteopath in question, at the end of that shorter period.

(6) In dealing with an application for registration made during the transitional period by a person who –

(a) cannot meet the requirement of subsection (2)(d), but

(b) has a qualification in osteopathy which, while not being a recognised qualification, has not been refused recognition by the General Council,

the Registrar shall refer the matter to the Education Committee.

(7) Where a reference is made to the Education Committee under subsection (6), it shall be the duty of the Committee to advise the General Council.

(8) If, after considering the advice of the Education Committee, the General Council is satisfied that it is appropriate to do so, it shall direct the Registrar to disregard subsection (2)(d) in relation to the application in question.

(9) For the purposes of subsection (2)(d), the question whether the applicant has spent any part of his working time in the lawful, safe and competent practice of osteopathy shall be determined in accordance with such rules (if any) as may be made by the General Council.

(10) In this section –

"required undertaking" means an undertaking that the person giving it will, before the end of the period of five years beginning with the opening of the register or such shorter period as the Registrar may specify in relation to the applicant –

(a) complete such additional training and acquire such experience as may be specified by the Registrar in accordance with rules made by the General Council; and

(b) comply with such other conditions (if any) as may be imposed on him by the Registrar in accordance with such rules; and

"transitional period" means the period of two years beginning with the opening of the register.

(11) Rules made by virtue of paragraph (b) in the definition of "required undertaking" in subsection (10) may, in particular, provide for the Registrar to be able to impose, as a condition, the passing of a test of competence specified by the Registrar.

Provisional registration.   **5.** – (1) The General Council may make rules providing for all applicants for registration who are entitled to be registered with full registration, or all such applicants falling within a prescribed class, to be registered initially with provisional registration.

(2) No such rules shall be made before the end of the period of two years beginning with the opening of the register.

(3) Before making any rules under subsection (1), the General Council shall take such steps as are reasonably practicable to consult those who are registered osteopaths.

(4) The General Council may by rules provide for the conversion, in prescribed circumstances and subject to the osteopath concerned complying with such conditions (if any) as may be prescribed, of provisional registration into full registration.

(5) Unless it is converted into full registration in accordance with the rules, any provisional registration shall cease to have effect at the end of the period of one year beginning with the date on which it is entered in the register.

(6) A provisionally registered osteopath shall not practise osteopathy except under the supervision of a fully registered osteopath who is approved by the General Council for the purposes of this subsection.

(7) The General Council shall maintain a list of those fully registered osteopaths who are for the time being approved by the Council for the purposes of subsection (6).

Registration: supplemental provision.

6. – (1) The register shall show, in relation to each registered osteopath –

(a)   whether he is registered with full, conditional or provisional registration; and

(b)   the address at which he has his practice or principal practice or, if he is not practising, such address as may be prescribed.

(2) The General Council may make rules in connection with registration and the register and as to the payment of fees.

(3) The rules may, in particular, make provision as to –

(a)   the form and keeping of the register;

(b)   the form and manner in which applications for registration are to be made;

(c)   the documentary and other evidence which is to accompany applications for registration;

(d)   the manner in which the Registrar is to satisfy himself as to the good character and competence of any person applying for registration and the procedure for so doing;

(e)   the manner in which the Registrar is to satisfy himself as to the physical and mental health of any person applying for registration and the procedure for so doing;

(f)   the description of persons from whom references are to be provided for persons applying for registration;

(g)   in the case of an application for conditional registration, the conditions or kinds of condition which may be imposed on the osteopath concerned;

(h) the making, periodic renewal and removal of entries in the register;

(i) the giving of reasons for any removal of, or refusal to renew, an entry in the register;

(j) any failure on the part of a registered osteopath to comply with any conditions subject to which his registration has effect, including provision for the Registrar to refuse to renew his registration or for the removal of his name from the register;

(k) the issue and form of certificates;

(l) the content, assessment and conduct of any test of competence imposed under section 4;

(m) the meaning of "principal practice" for the purposes of subsection (1).

(4) The rules may, in particular, also make provision –

(a) prescribing the fee to be charged for making an entry in the register or restoring such an entry;

(b) prescribing the fee to be charged in respect of the retention in the register of any entry in any year following the year in which the entry was first made;

(c) providing for the entry in the register of qualifications (whether or not they are recognised qualifications) possessed by registered osteopaths and the removal of such an entry;

(d) prescribing the fee to be charged in respect of the making or removal of any entry of a kind mentioned in paragraph (c);

(e) authorising the Registrar –

(i) to refuse to make an entry in the register, or restore such an entry, until the prescribed fee has been paid;

(ii) to remove from the register any entry relating to a person who, after the prescribed notice has been given, fails to pay the fee prescribed in respect of the retention of the entry.

(5) A person who has failed to renew his registration as an osteopath shall be entitled to have his entry restored to the register on payment of the prescribed fee.

Suspension of registration.

7. – (1) Where the Registrar suspends the registration of an osteopath in accordance with any provision of this Act, the Registrar shall enter in the register a note of –

(a) the suspension;

(b) the period of the suspension; and

(c) the provision under which the suspension was made.

(2) Where the period of the suspension is extended, the Registrar shall note the extension in the register.

(3) Any osteopath whose registration has been suspended shall, for the period of his suspension, cease to be a registered osteopath for the purposes of section 32(1).

Restoration to the register of osteopaths who have been struck off.

8. – (1) Where a person who has had his entry as a fully registered osteopath removed from the register as the result of an order under section 22(4)(d) wishes to have his entry restored to the register he shall make an application for registration to the Registrar.

(2) No such application may be made before the end of the period of ten months beginning with the date on which the order under section 22(4)(d) was made.

(3) Any application for registration in the circumstances mentioned in subsection (1) (an "application for restoration") shall be referred by the Registrar to the Professional Conduct Committee for determination by that Committee.

(4) For the purposes of determining an application for restoration –

(a) the Committee shall exercise the Registrar's functions under section 3; and

(b) subsection (2) of that section shall have effect as if paragraph (d) were omitted.

(5) The Committee shall not grant an application for restoration unless it is satisfied that the applicant not only satisfies the requirements of section 3 (as modified) but, having regard in particular to the circumstances which led to the making of the order under section 22(4)(d), is also a fit and proper person to practise the profession of osteopathy.

(6) On granting an application for restoration, the Committee –

(a) shall direct the Registrar to register the applicant as a fully registered osteopath; and

(b) may make a conditions of practice order with respect to him.

(7) The provisions of section 22 shall have effect in relation to a conditions of practice order made by virtue of subsection (6) as they have effect in relation to one made by virtue of subsection (4)(b) of that section.

(8) The General Council may by rules make provision in relation to the restoration to the register of conditionally registered osteopaths or provisionally registered osteopaths, and any such rules may provide for restoration, in prescribed circumstances, as a fully registered osteopath.

Access to the register etc.

9. – (1) The General Council shall –

(a)   make the register available for inspection by members of the public at all reasonable times; and

(b)   publish the register before the end of the period of twelve months beginning with the opening of the register and at least once in every succeeding period of twelve months.

(2) Any person who asks the General Council for a copy of the most recently published register shall be entitled to have one on payment of such reasonable fee as the Council may determine.

(3) Subsection (2) shall not be taken as preventing the General Council from providing copies of the register free of charge whenever it considers it appropriate.

(4) Any copy of, or extract from, the published register shall be evidence (and in Scotland sufficient evidence) of the matters mentioned in it.

(5) A certificate purporting to be signed by the Registrar, certifying that a person –

(a)   is registered in a specified category,

(b)   is not registered,

(c)   was registered in a specified category at a specified date or during a specified period,

(d)   was not registered in a specified category, or in any category, at a specified date or during a specified period, or

(e)   has never been registered,

shall be evidence (and in Scotland sufficient evidence) of the matters certified.

Fraud or error in
relation to
registration.

10. – (1) The Registrar shall investigate any allegation that an entry in the register has been fraudulently procured or incorrectly made and report on the result of his investigation to the General Council.

(2) An entry which has been restored to the register under section 6(5) or section 8, or under rules made by virtue of section 8(8), may be treated for the purposes of this section as having been fraudulently procured or incorrectly made if any previous entry from which the restored entry is derived was fraudulently procured or incorrectly made.

(3) The Registrar may, at any time during his investigation, suspend the registration in question if he is satisfied that it is necessary to do so in order to protect members of the public.

(4) The General Council shall by rules make provision, in relation to any case where the Registrar proposes to suspend an osteopath's registration under subsection (3) –

(a) giving the osteopath concerned an opportunity to appear before the Investigating Committee and argue his case against suspension;

(b) allowing him to be legally represented; and

(c) for the Registrar to be made a party to the proceedings.

(5) If, having considered any report of the Registrar, the General Council is satisfied that the entry in question has been fraudulently procured or incorrectly made it may order the Registrar to remove the entry.

(6) Where such an order is made, the Registrar shall without delay notify the person whose entry is to be removed –

(a) of the order; and

(b) of the right of appeal given by subsection (7).

(7) Where such an order is made, the person whose entry is to be removed may appeal to Her Majesty in Council.

(8) Any such appeal –

(a) must be brought before the end of the period of 28 days beginning with the date on which the order is made; and

(b) shall be dealt with in accordance with rules made by Her Majesty by Order in Council for the purposes of this section.

(9) On an appeal under this section, the General Council shall be the respondent.

(10) The [1833 c. 41.] Judicial Committee Act 1833 shall apply in relation to the General Council as it applies in relation to any court from which an appeal lies to Her Majesty in Council.

(11) Without prejudice to the application of that Act, on an appeal under this section to Her Majesty in Council the Judicial Committee may, in their report, recommend to Her Majesty in Council –

(a) that the appeal be dismissed; or

(b) that it be allowed and the order appealed against quashed.

(12) The General Council may by rules make such further provision as it considers appropriate with respect to suspensions under subsection (3), including in particular provision as to their duration.

Professional education

The Education
Committee.

11. – (1) The Education Committee shall have the general duty of promoting high standards of education and training in osteopathy and keeping the provision made for that education and training under review.

(2) Where it considers it to be necessary in connection with the discharge of its general duty, the Education Committee may itself provide, or arrange for the provision of, education or training.

(3) The General Council shall consult the Education Committee on matters relating to education, training, examinations or tests of competence.

(4) It shall be the duty of the Education Committee to give advice to the General Council on the matters mentioned in subsection (3), either on being consulted by the Council or where it considers it appropriate to do so.

Visitors.

12. – (1) The Education Committee may appoint persons to visit any place at which or institution by which or under whose direction –

(a) any relevant course of study is, or is proposed to be, given;

(b) any examination is, or is proposed to be, held in connection with any such course;

(c) any test of competence is, or is proposed to be, conducted in connection with any such course or for any other purpose connected with this Act.

(2) In subsection (1) "relevant course of study" means any course of study which forms, or is intended to form, part of –

(a) the complete course of study required in order to obtain a recognised qualification or a qualification for which recognition is being sought; or

(b) any training which a registered osteopath may be required to undergo after registration.

(3) No person appointed as a visitor may exercise his functions under this section in relation to –

(a) any place at which he regularly gives instruction in any subject; or

(b) any institution with which he has a significant connection.

(4) A person shall not be prevented from being appointed as a visitor merely because he is a member of –

(a) the General Council; or

(b) any of its committees.

(5) Where a visitor visits any place or institution, in the exercise of his functions under this section, he shall report to the Education Committee –

(a) on the nature and quality of the instruction given, or to be given, and the facilities provided or to be provided, at that place or by that institution; and

(b) on such other matters (if any) as he was required to report on by the Committee.

(6) Requirements of the kind mentioned in subsection (5)(b) may be imposed by the Education Committee –

(a) generally in relation to all visits;

(b) generally in relation to all visits made to a specified kind of place or institution; or

(c) specifically in relation to a particular visit.

(7) Where a visitor reports to the Education Committee under subsection (5), the Committee shall on receipt of the report –

(a) send a copy of it to the institution concerned; and

(b) notify that institution of the period within which it may make observations on, or raise objections to, the report.

(8) The period specified by the Committee in a notice given under subsection (7)(b) shall not be less than one month beginning with the date on which a copy of the report is sent to the institution under subsection (7)(a).

(9) The Education Committee shall not take any steps in the light of any report made under subsection (5) before the end of the specified period.

(10) The General Council may –

(a) pay fees, allowances and expenses to persons appointed as visitors; or

(b) treat any such person, for the purposes of paragraph 15(2)(c) to (e) of the Schedule, as a member of its staff.

(11) In the case of a visitor who is also such a member as is mentioned in subsection (4), any payment made to him in his capacity as a visitor shall be in addition to any to which he is entitled as such a member.

The standard of proficiency.

13. – (1) The General Council shall from time to time determine the standard of proficiency which, in its opinion, is required for the competent and safe practice of osteopathy.

(2) The Council shall publish a statement of the standard of proficiency determined by it under this section.

(3) If the Council at any time varies the standard so determined it shall publish –

(a) a statement of the revised standard; and

(b) a statement of the differences between that standard and the standard as it was immediately before the revision.

(4) No variation of the standard shall have effect before the end of the period of one year beginning with the date on which the Council publishes the statement required by subsection (3) in connection with that variation.

Recognition of qualifications.

14. – (1) For the purposes of this Act, a qualification is a "recognised qualification" if it is recognised by the General Council under this section.

(2) Where the General Council is satisfied that –

(a) a qualification granted by an institution in the United Kingdom is evidence of having reached the required standard of proficiency, or

(b) a qualification which such an institution proposes to grant will be evidence of having reached that standard,

it may, with the approval of the Privy Council, recognise that qualification for the purposes of this Act.

(3) Where the General Council is satisfied that a qualification granted by an institution outside the United Kingdom is evidence of having reached the required standard of proficiency, or of reaching a comparable standard, it may, with the approval of the Privy Council, recognise that qualification for the purposes of this Act.

(4) The General Council may by rules –

(a) impose additional conditions for registration, or

(b) provide for any provision made by this Act in relation to conditions for registration to have effect subject to prescribed modifications,

in the case of any application for registration based on a person's holding a qualification which is recognised under subsection (3).

(5) The General Council shall maintain and publish a list of the qualifications which are for the time being recognised under this section.

(6) Before deciding whether or not to recognise a qualification under this section, the General Council shall consult the Education Committee.

(7) When requesting the approval of the Privy Council for the purposes of subsection (2) or (3), the General Council shall make available to the Privy Council –

(a) the information provided to it by the Education Committee; or

(b) where the Privy Council considers it appropriate, a summary of that information.

(8) The Privy Council shall have regard to the information made available to it under subsection (7) before deciding whether or not to give its approval.

(9) The General Council may by rules make provision requiring the Education Committee to publish a statement indicating –

(a) matters on which the Committee will wish to be satisfied before advising the General Council to recognise a qualification under subsection (2); and

(b) matters which may cause the Committee to advise the General Council not to recognise a qualification under subsection (2).

(10) Where, by virtue of Community law a person ("the osteopath") is to be authorised to practise the profession of osteopathy on the same conditions as a person who holds a recognised qualification –

(a) the osteopath shall be treated for the purposes of this Act as having a recognised qualification; but

(b) the General Council may, subject to Community law, require him to satisfy specified additional conditions before being registered.

(11) In subsection (10) "Community law" means any enforceable Community right or any enactment giving effect to a Community obligation.

Recognition of qualifications: supplemental.

15. – (1) A qualification may be recognised by the General Council under section 14 –

(a) only in respect of awards of that qualification made after a specified date;

(b) only in respect of awards made before a specified date; or

(c) only in respect of awards made after a specified date but before a specified date.

(2) Any date specified under subsection (1) may be earlier than the date on which this Act is passed.

(3) Where the General Council recognises a qualification in one or other of the limited ways allowed for by subsection (1), the limitation shall be specified in the list issued by the Council under section 14(5).

(4) The General Council may, in recognising a qualification under section 14, direct that the qualification is to remain a recognised qualification only so long as such conditions as the General Council sees fit to impose are complied with in relation to the qualification.

(5) Any such condition may at any time be removed by the General Council.

(6) The General Council shall not exercise any of its functions under subsection (4) or (5) without the approval of the Privy Council.

(7) Any institution which is, or is likely to be, affected by a direction given by the General Council under subsection (4) shall be notified by the Council of the direction as soon as is reasonably practicable.

(8) Where an application is made by any institution for the recognition of a qualification under section 14, the General Council shall notify the institution of the result of its application as soon as is reasonably practicable after the Council determines the application.

(9) Where the General Council refuses such an application it shall, when notifying the institution concerned, give reasons for its refusal.

Withdrawal of recognition.

16. – (1) Where, as a result of any visitor's report or other information acquired by the Education Committee, the Committee is of the opinion –

(a)   that a recognised qualification is no longer, or will no longer be, evidence of having reached the required standard of proficiency,

(b)   that a proposed qualification which has yet to be granted, but which was recognised by virtue of section 14(2)(b), will not be evidence of having reached that standard, or

(c)   that a condition for the continued recognition of a qualification (imposed under section 15(4)) has not been complied with,

it shall refer the matter to the General Council.

(2) If the General Council is satisfied that the circumstances of the case are as mentioned in subsection (1)(a), (b) or (c) it may, with the approval of the Privy Council, direct that the qualification is no longer to be a recognised qualification for the purposes of this Act.

(3) A direction under subsection (2) shall have effect from the date of the direction or from such later date as may be specified in the direction.

(4) In considering any matter referred to it under subsection (1), the General Council shall have regard to the information on which the Education Committee formed its opinion together with any other relevant information which the Council may have.

(5) When requesting the approval of the Privy Council for the purposes of subsection (2), the General Council shall make available to the Privy Council the information to which it had regard under subsection (4).

(6) The Privy Council shall have regard to the information made available to it under subsection (5) before deciding whether or not to give its approval.

(7) Where the recognition of any qualification is withdrawn under this section, the General Council shall use its best endeavours to secure that any person who is studying for that qualification at any place, at the time when recognition is withdrawn, is given the opportunity to study at that or any other place for a qualification which is recognised.

(8) The withdrawal under this section of recognition from any qualification shall not affect the entitlement of any person to be registered by reference to an award of that qualification made to him before the date on which the direction withdrawing recognition had effect.

Post registration training.

17. – (1) The General Council may make rules requiring registered osteopaths to undertake further courses of training.

(2) The rules may, in particular, make provision with respect to registered osteopaths who fail to comply with any requirements of the rules, including provision for their registration to cease to have effect.

(3) Before making, or varying, any rules under this section the General Council shall take such steps as are reasonably practicable to consult those who are registered osteopaths and such other persons as the Council considers appropriate.

Information to be given by institutions.

18. – (1) This section applies to any institution by which, or under whose direction –

    (a) any relevant course of study is, or is proposed to be, given;

    (b) any examination is, or is proposed to be, held in connection with any such course; or

    (c) any test of competence is, or is proposed to be, conducted in connection with any such course or for any other purpose connected with this Act.

(2) In subsection (1) "relevant course of study" has the same meaning as in section 12.

(3) Whenever required to do so by the General Council, any such institution shall give to the Council such information as the Council may reasonably require in connection with the exercise of its functions under this Act.

(4) The matters with respect to which the General Council may require information under subsection (3) include –

(a) the requirements which must be met by any person pursuing the course of study, undergoing the course of training or taking the examination or test in question;

(b) the financial position of the institution;

(c) the efficiency of the institution's management.

(5) Where an institution refuses any reasonable request for information made by the General Council under this section, the Council may on that ground alone –

(a) give a direction under section 16(2) (with the required approval of the Privy Council) in respect of the qualification in question; or

(b) refuse to recognise that qualification under section 14.

Professional conduct and fitness to practise

The Code of Practice.   **19.** – (1) The General Council shall prepare and from time to time publish a Code of Practice –

(a) laying down standards of conduct and practice expected of registered osteopaths; and

(b) giving advice in relation to the practice of osteopathy.

(2) It shall be the duty of the General Council to keep the Code under review and to vary its provisions whenever the Council considers it appropriate to do so.

(3) Before issuing the Code or varying it, the General Council shall consult such representatives of practising osteopaths as it considers appropriate.

(4) Where any person is alleged to have failed to comply with any provision of the Code, that failure –

(a) shall not be taken, of itself, to constitute unacceptable professional conduct on his part; but

(b) shall be taken into account in any proceedings against him under this Act.

(5) Any person who asks the General Council for a copy of the Code shall be entitled to have one on payment of such reasonable fee as the Council may determine.

(6) Subsection (5) is not to be taken as preventing the General Council from providing copies of the Code free of charge whenever it considers it appropriate.

Professional conduct and fitness to practise.

20. – (1) This section applies where any allegation is made against a registered osteopath to the effect that –

(a) he has been guilty of conduct which falls short of the standard required of a registered osteopath;

(b) he has been guilty of professional incompetence;

(c) he has been convicted (at any time) in the United Kingdom of a criminal offence; or

(d) his ability to practise as an osteopath is seriously impaired because of his physical or mental condition.

(2) In this Act conduct which falls short of the standard required of a registered osteopath is referred to as "unacceptable professional conduct".

(3) Where an allegation is made to the General Council, or to any of its committees (other than the Investigating Committee), it shall be the duty of the Council or committee to refer the allegation to the Investigating Committee.

(4) The General Council may make rules requiring any allegation which is made or referred to the Investigating Committee to be referred for preliminary consideration to a person appointed by the Council in accordance with the rules.

(5) Any rules made under subsection (4) –

(a) may allow for the appointment of persons who are members of the General Council; but

(b) may not allow for the appointment of the Registrar.

(6) Any person to whom an allegation is referred by the Investigating Committee in accordance with rules made under subsection (4) shall –

(a) consider the allegation with a view to establishing whether, in his opinion, power is given by this Act to deal with it if it proves to be well founded; and

(b) if he considers that such power is given, give the Investigating Committee a report of the result of his consideration.

(7) Where there are rules in force under subsection (4), the Investigating Committee shall investigate any allegation with respect to which it is given a report by a person appointed under the rules.

(8) Where there are no such rules in force, the Investigating Committee shall investigate any allegation which is made or referred to it.

(9) Where the Investigating Committee is required to investigate any allegation, it shall –

(a) notify the registered osteopath concerned of the allegation and invite him to give it his observations before the end of the period of 28 days beginning with the day on which notice of the allegation is sent to him;

(b) take such steps as are reasonably practicable to obtain as much information as possible about the case; and

(c) consider, in the light of the information which it has been able to obtain and any observations duly made to it by the registered osteopath concerned, whether in its opinion there is a case to answer.

(10) The General Council may by rules make provision as to the procedure to be followed by the Investigating Committee in any investigation carried out by it under this section.

(11) In the case of an allegation of a kind mentioned in subsection (1)(c), the Investigating Committee may conclude that there is no case to answer if it considers that the criminal offence in question has no material relevance to the fitness of the osteopath concerned to practise osteopathy.

(12) Where the Investigating Committee concludes that there is a case to answer, it shall –

(a) notify both the osteopath concerned and the person making the allegation of its conclusion; and

(b) refer the allegation, as formulated by the Investigating Committee –

(i) to the Health Committee, in the case of an allegation of a kind mentioned in subsection (1)(d); or

(ii) to the Professional Conduct Committee, in the case of an allegation of any other kind.

(13) Where the Investigating Committee concludes that there is no case to answer, it shall notify both the osteopath concerned and the person making the allegation.

(14) In this section "allegation" means an allegation of a kind mentioned in subsection (1).

Interim suspension powers of the Investigating Committee.

21. – (1) This section applies where, under section 20, the Investigating Committee is investigating an allegation against a registered osteopath.

(2) If the Committee is satisfied that it is necessary to do so in order to protect members of the public, it may order the Registrar to suspend the osteopath's registration.

(3) The order shall specify the period of the suspension, which shall not exceed two months beginning with the date on which the order is made.

(4) The Committee shall not –

(a) make an order in any case after it has referred the allegation in question to the Professional Conduct Committee or the Health Committee; or

(b) make more than one order in respect of the same allegation.

(5) Before making an order, the Investigating Committee shall give the osteopath concerned an opportunity to appear before it and to argue his case against the making of the proposed order.

(6) At any such hearing the osteopath shall be entitled to be legally represented.

Consideration of allegations by the Professional Conduct Committee.

22. – (1) Where an allegation has been referred to the Professional Conduct Committee under section 20 or by virtue of any rule made under section 26(2)(a), it shall be the duty of the Committee to consider the allegation.

(2) If, having considered it, the Committee is satisfied that the allegation is well founded it shall proceed as follows.

(3) If the allegation is of a kind mentioned in section 20(1)(c), the Committee may take no further action if it considers that the criminal offence in question has no material relevance to the fitness of the osteopath concerned to practise osteopathy.

(4) Otherwise, the Committee shall take one of the following steps –

(a) admonish the osteopath;

(b) make an order imposing conditions with which he must comply while practising as an osteopath (a "conditions of practice order");

(c) order the Registrar to suspend the osteopath's registration for such period as may be specified in the order (a "suspension order"); or

(d) order the Registrar to remove the osteopath's name from the register.

(5) A conditions of practice order shall cease to have effect –

(a) if a period is specified in the order for the purposes of this subsection, when that period ends;

(b) if no such period is specified but a test of competence is so specified, when the osteopath concerned passes the test; or

(c) if both a period and a test are so specified, when the period ends or when the osteopath concerned passes the test, whichever is the later to occur.

(6) At any time while a conditions of practice order is in force under this section or by virtue of a recommendation under section 31(8)(c), the Committee may (whether or not of its own motion) –

(a) extend, or further extend, the period for which the order has effect;

(b) revoke or vary any of the conditions;

(c) require the osteopath concerned to pass a test of competence specified by the Committee;

(d) reduce the period for which the order has effect; or

(e) revoke the order.

(7) Where the period for which a conditions of practice order has effect is extended or reduced under subsection (6), or a test of competence is specified under that subsection, subsection (5) shall have effect as if –

(a) the period specified in the conditions of practice order was the extended or reduced period; and

(b) the test of competence was specified in that order.

(8) At any time while a suspension order is in force with respect to an osteopath under this section or by virtue of a recommendation under section 31(8)(c), the Committee may (whether or not of its own motion) –

(a) extend, or further extend, the period of suspension; and

(b) make a conditions of practice order with which the osteopath must comply if he resumes the practice of osteopathy after the end of his period of suspension.

(9) The period specified in a conditions of practice order or in a suspension order under this section, and any extension of a specified period under subsection (6) or (8), shall not in each case exceed three years.

(10) Before exercising its powers under subsection (4), (6) or (8), the Committee shall give the osteopath concerned an opportunity to appear before it and to argue his case.

(11) At any such hearing the osteopath shall be entitled to be legally represented.

(12) In exercising its powers under subsection (6) or (8), the Committee shall ensure that the conditions imposed on the osteopath concerned are, or the period of suspension imposed on him is, the minimum which it considers necessary for the protection of members of the public.

(13) The Committee shall, before the end of the period of twelve months beginning with the commencement of this section, and at least once in every succeeding period of twelve months, publish a report setting out –

(a) the names of those osteopaths in respect of whom it has investigated allegations under this section and found the allegations to be well founded;

(b) the nature of those allegations; and

(c) the steps (if any) taken by the Committee in respect of the osteopaths so named.

(14) Where the Committee has investigated any allegation against an osteopath under this section and has not been satisfied that the allegation was well founded, it shall include in its report for the year in question a statement of that fact if the osteopath so requests.

Consideration of **23.** – (1) Where an allegation has been referred to the Health
allegations by the Committee under section 20 or by virtue of any rule made under
Health Committee. section 26(2)(a), it shall be the duty of the Committee to consider the
allegation.

(2) If, having considered it, the Committee is satisfied that the
allegation is well founded, it shall –

(a) make an order imposing conditions with which the
osteopath concerned must comply while practising as an
osteopath (a "conditions of practice order"); or

(b) order the Registrar to suspend the osteopath's registration
for such period as may be specified in the order (a "suspension
order").

(3) Any condition in a conditions of practice order under this section
shall be imposed so as to have effect for a period specified in the order.

(4) At any time while a conditions of practice order is in force under
this section or under section 30 or by virtue of a recommendation
under section 31(8)(c), the Committee may (whether or not of its
own motion) –

(a) extend, or further extend, the period for which the order
has effect; or

(b) make a suspension order with respect to the osteopath
concerned.

(5) At any time while a suspension order is in force with respect to
an osteopath under this section or under section 30 or by virtue of a
recommendation under section 31(8)(c), the Committee may
(whether or not of its own motion) –

(a) extend, or further extend, the period of suspension;

(b) replace the order with a conditions of practice order having
effect for the remainder of the period of suspension; or

(c) make a conditions of practice order with which the
osteopath must comply if he resumes the practice of osteopathy
after the end of his period of suspension.

(6) On the application of the osteopath with respect to whom a
conditions of practice order or a suspension order is in force under this
section or under section 30 or by virtue of a recommendation under
section 31(8)(c), the Committee may –

(a) revoke the order;

(b) vary the order by reducing the period for which it has effect; or

(c) in the case of a conditions of practice order, vary the order by removing or altering any of the conditions.

(7) Where an osteopath has made an application under subsection (6) which has been refused ("the previous application"), the Committee shall not entertain a further such application unless it is made after the end of the period of twelve months beginning with the date on which the previous application was received by the Committee.

(8) The period specified in a conditions of practice order or in a suspension order under this section, and any extension of a specified period under subsection (4) or (5), shall not in each case exceed three years.

(9) Before exercising its powers under subsection (2), (4), (5) or (6), the Committee shall give the osteopath concerned an opportunity to appear before it and to argue his case.

(10) At any such hearing the osteopath shall be entitled to be legally represented.

(11) In exercising any of its powers under this section, the Committee shall ensure that any conditions imposed on the osteopath concerned are, or any period of suspension imposed on him is, the minimum which it considers necessary for the protection of members of the public.

Interim suspension powers of the Professional Conduct Committee and the Health Committee.

24. – (1) This section applies where –

(a) an allegation against a registered osteopath has been referred under section 20, or by virtue of any rule made under section 26(2)(a), to the Professional Conduct Committee or the Health Committee and the Committee has not reached a decision on the matter; or

(b) the Professional Conduct Committee or the Health Committee reaches a relevant decision on any such allegation.

(2) The Committee concerned may, if it is satisfied that it is necessary to do so in order to protect members of the public, order the Registrar to suspend the registration of the osteopath concerned.

(3) An order under subsection (2) (an "interim suspension order") shall cease to have effect –

(a) in a case falling within subsection (1)(a), when the Committee reaches a decision in respect of the allegation in question; and

(b) in a case falling within subsection (1)(b) –

(i) if there is no appeal against the decision, when the period for appealing expires; or

(ii) if there is an appeal against the decision, when the appeal is withdrawn or otherwise disposed of.

(4) Before making an interim suspension order, the Committee shall give the osteopath in question an opportunity to appear before it and to argue his case against the making of the proposed order.

(5) At any such hearing the osteopath shall be entitled to be legally represented.

(6) Where an interim suspension order has been made, the osteopath concerned may appeal against it to the appropriate court.

(7) Any such appeal must be brought before the end of the period of 28 days beginning with the date on which the order appealed against is made.

(8) On an appeal under subsection (6) the court may terminate the suspension.

(9) On such an appeal the decision of the court shall be final.

(10) In this section –

"the appropriate court" means –

(a) in the case of an osteopath whose registered address is in Scotland, the Court of Session;

(b) in the case of an osteopath whose registered address is in Northern Ireland, the High Court of Justice in Northern Ireland; and

(c) in any other case, the High Court of Justice in England and Wales;

"relevant decision" means an order under section 22(4)(c) or (d), or an order under section 23(2)(b).

Revocation of interim suspension orders.

25. – (1) On an application made by the osteopath concerned, in a case falling within section 24(1)(a), an interim suspension order may be revoked by the Committee which made it on the ground that a change in the circumstances of the case has made the order unnecessary.

(2) Where an osteopath has made an application under subsection (1) which has been refused, he may appeal to the appropriate court against the refusal.

(3) Where, in relation to an interim suspension order –

(a) an appeal has been made under section 24(6) against the making of the order, or

(b) a further application for the order to be revoked has been made after an unsuccessful appeal under this section against the refusal of an earlier application,

leave of the appropriate court shall be required for any appeal under subsection (2) in relation to that order.

(4) Except in a case falling within subsection (5), no application under subsection (1) shall be entertained by the Committee concerned if it is made before the end of the period of six months beginning –

(a) with the date on which the order was imposed; or

(b) where an unsuccessful appeal against the order has been made under section 24(6), the date on which the appeal was dismissed.

(5) Where a previous application has been made under subsection (1) in relation to an interim suspension order, no further such application shall be entertained by the Committee concerned if it is made before the end of the period of six months beginning with the date on which the previous application was finally disposed of.

(6) Any appeal under subsection (2) must be brought before the end of the period of 28 days beginning with the date on which notice of the refusal is sent to the osteopath.

(7) On an appeal under subsection (2) the court may terminate the suspension.

(8) On such an appeal the decision of the court shall be final.

(9) In this section "the appropriate court" has the same meaning as in section 24.

Investigation of allegations: procedural rules.

26. – (1) The General Council shall make rules as to the procedure to be followed by the Professional Conduct Committee or the Health Committee in considering any allegation under section 22 or 23.

(2) The rules shall, in particular, include provision –

(a) empowering each Committee to refer to the other any allegation which it considers would be better dealt with by that other Committee;

(b) requiring the osteopath to whom the allegation relates to be given notice of the allegation;

(c) giving the osteopath an opportunity to put his case at a hearing if –

(i) before the end of the period of 28 days beginning with the date on which notice of the allegation is sent to him, he asks for a hearing; or

(ii) the Committee considers that a hearing is desirable;

(d) entitling the osteopath to be legally represented at any hearing in respect of the allegation;

(e) securing that –

(i) any hearing before the Professional Conduct Committee is held in public unless the Committee decides that it is in the interests of the person making the allegation, or of any person giving evidence or of any patient, to hold the hearing or any part of it in private; and

(ii) any hearing before the Health Committee is held in private unless the Committee considers that it is appropriate to hold the hearing or any part of it in public;

(f) requiring the osteopath to be notified by the Committee of its decision, its reasons for reaching that decision and of his right of appeal;

(g) requiring the person by whom the allegation was made to be notified by the Committee of its decision and of its reasons for reaching that decision;

(h) empowering the Committee to require persons to attend and give evidence or to produce documents;

(i)   about the admissibility of evidence;

(j)   enabling the Committee to administer oaths.

(3) No person shall be required by any rules made under this section to give any evidence or produce any document or other material at a

hearing held by either Committee which he could not be compelled to give or produce in civil proceedings in any court in that part of the United Kingdom in which the hearing takes place.

Legal assessors.

27. – (1) The General Council shall appoint persons to be legal assessors.

(2) They shall have the general function of giving advice to –

(a) any person appointed in accordance with rules made under section 20(4),

(b) the Investigating Committee,

(c) the Professional Conduct Committee, or

(d) the Health Committee,

on questions of law arising in connection with any matter which he or (as the case may be) the committee is considering.

(3) They shall also have such other functions as may be conferred on them by rules made by the General Council.

(4) To be qualified for appointment as a legal assessor under this section, a person must –

(a) have a 10 year general qualification (within the meaning of section 71 of the [1990 c. 41.] Courts and Legal Services Act 1990);

(b) be an advocate or solicitor in Scotland of at least 10 years' standing; or

(c) be a member of the Bar of Northern Ireland or solicitor of the Supreme Court of Northern Ireland of at least 10 years' standing.

(5) The General Council may pay such fees, allowances and expenses to persons appointed as legal assessors as it may determine.

(6) In the case of a legal assessor who is also a member of the General Council or of any of its committees, any such payment made to him in his capacity as a legal assessor shall be in addition to any to which he is entitled as such a member.

Medical assessors.

28. – (1) The General Council may appoint registered medical practitioners to be medical assessors.

(2) They shall have the general function of giving advice to –

(a) any person appointed in accordance with rules made under section 20(4),

(b) the Investigating Committee,

(c) the Professional Conduct Committee, or

(d) the Health Committee,

on matters within their professional competence arising in connection with any matter which he or (as the case may be) the committee is considering.

(3) They shall also have such other functions as may be conferred on them by rules made by the General Council.

(4) The General Council may pay such fees, allowances and expenses to persons appointed as medical assessors as it may determine.

(5) In the case of a medical assessor who is also a member of the General Council or of any of its committees, any such payment made to him in his capacity as a medical assessor shall be in addition to any to which he is entitled as such a member.

Appeals

Appeals against decisions of the Registrar.

29. – (1) Where the Registrar –

(a) refuses to register an applicant for registration under this Act,

(b) registers such an applicant with provisional or conditional registration,

(c) refuses to renew any registration,

(d) removes the name of a registered osteopath from the register on the ground that he has breached one or more of the conditions subject to which his registration had effect (otherwise than under an order of the Professional Conduct Committee), or

(e) refuses to grant an application for the conversion of a conditional, or provisional, registration into full registration,

the person aggrieved may appeal to the General Council.

(2) Any such appeal shall be subject to such rules as the General Council may make for the purpose of regulating appeals under this section.

(3) An appeal to the General Council must be made before the end of the period of 28 days beginning with the date on which notice of the Registrar's decision is sent to the person concerned.

(4) Any person aggrieved by the decision of the General Council on an appeal under this section may appeal, on a point of law, to the appropriate court.

(5) Any right of appeal given by this section shall be in addition to any right which the person concerned may otherwise have to appeal to a county court or, in Scotland, to the sheriff; but only one such right of appeal may be exercised in relation to the same decision.

(6) In this section "the appropriate court" means –

(a) in the case of a person whose registered address is (or if he were registered would be) in Scotland, the Court of Session;

(b) in the case of a person whose registered address is (or if he were registered would be) in Northern Ireland, the High Court of Justice in Northern Ireland; and

(c) in any other case, the High Court of Justice in England and Wales.

Appeals against decisions of the Health Committee.
30. – (1) Any person with respect to whom a decision of the Health Committee is made under section 23 may, before the end of the period of 28 days beginning with the date on which notification of the decision is sent to him, appeal against it in accordance with the provisions of this section.

(2) An appeal under subsection (1) shall lie to an appeal tribunal, consisting of a chairman and two other members, established for the purposes of the appeal in accordance with rules made by the General Council for the purposes of this section.

(3) The General Council shall make rules as to the procedure to be followed by an appeal tribunal hearing an appeal under this section.

(4) The rules may, in particular, make similar provision to that made by virtue of section 26(2)(d), (f), (g), (h), (i) or (j).

(5) No decision against which an appeal may be made under this section shall have effect before –

(a) the expiry of the period within which such an appeal may be made; or

(b) the appeal is withdrawn or otherwise disposed of.

(6) The chairman of an appeal tribunal –

(a) shall be selected in accordance with rules made by the General Council; and

(b) shall be qualified as mentioned in section 27(4).

(7) Each of the other two members of an appeal tribunal shall be selected in accordance with rules made by the General Council –

(a) one of them being a fully registered osteopath, and

(b) the other being a registered medical practitioner.

(8) The rules may not provide for the selection of any member of an appeal tribunal to be by the General Council.

(9) The chairman of an appeal tribunal shall appoint a person approved by the members of the tribunal to act as clerk of the tribunal.

(10) Subject to any provision made by the rules, an appeal tribunal shall sit in public and shall sit –

(a) in Northern Ireland, in the case of an osteopath whose registered address is in Northern Ireland;

(b) in Scotland, in the case of an osteopath whose registered address is in Scotland; and

(c) in England and Wales, in any other case.

(11) On any appeal under this section –

(a) the appeal shall be by way of a rehearing of the case;

(b) the General Council shall be the respondent; and

(c) the tribunal hearing the appeal shall have power to make any decision which the Health Committee had power to make under section 23.

(12) An appeal tribunal shall have the same powers of interim suspension as the Health Committee has under section 24(1)(b) and that section shall have effect in relation to suspension orders made by appeal tribunals with the necessary modifications.

(13) No person shall be required by any rules made under this section to give any evidence or produce any document or other material at a hearing held by an appeal tribunal which he could not be

compelled to give or produce in civil proceedings in any court in that part of the United Kingdom in which the hearing takes place.

(14) An appeal tribunal shall have power to award costs.

(15) Any expenses reasonably incurred by a tribunal, including any incurred in connection with the appointment of a clerk, shall be met by the General Council.

Appeals against decisions of the Professional Conduct Committee and appeal tribunals.

31. – (1) Any person with respect to whom –

(a) a decision of the Professional Conduct Committee is made under section 22, or

(b) a decision is made by an appeal tribunal hearing an appeal under section 30,

may, before the end of the period of 28 days beginning with the date on which notification of the decision is sent to him, appeal against it in accordance with the provisions of this section.

(2) No such decision shall have effect –

(a) before the expiry of the period within which an appeal against the decision may be made; or

(b) where an appeal against the decision has been duly made, before the appeal is withdrawn or otherwise disposed of.

(3) An appeal under this section shall lie to Her Majesty in Council.

(4) An appeal under subsection (1)(b) may only be on a point of law.

(5) Any such appeal shall be dealt with in accordance with rules made by Her Majesty by Order in Council for the purposes of this section.

(6) On an appeal under this section, the General Council shall be the respondent.

(7) The [1833 c. 41.] Judicial Committee Act 1833 shall apply in relation to the Professional Conduct Committee, the Health Committee and the General Council as it applies in relation to any court from which an appeal lies to Her Majesty in Council.

(8) Without prejudice to the application of that Act, on an appeal under this section to Her Majesty in Council, the Judicial Committee may in their report recommend to Her Majesty in Council –

(a) that the appeal be dismissed;

(b) that the appeal be allowed and the decision questioned by the appeal quashed;

(c) that such other decision as the Professional Conduct Committee or (as the case may be) Health Committee could have made be substituted for the decision questioned by the appeal; or

(d) that the case be remitted to the Committee or appeal tribunal concerned to be disposed of in accordance with the directions of the Judicial Committee.

Offences

Offences.
32. – (1) A person who (whether expressly or by implication) describes himself as an osteopath, osteopathic practitioner, osteopathic physician, osteopathist, osteotherapist, or any other kind of osteopath, is guilty of an offence unless he is a registered osteopath.

(2) A person who, without reasonable excuse, fails to comply with any requirement imposed by –

(a) the Professional Conduct Committee,

(b) the Health Committee, or

(c) an appeal tribunal hearing an appeal under section 30,

under rules made by virtue of section 26(2)(h) or under any corresponding rules made by virtue of section 30(4) is guilty of an offence.

(3) A person guilty of an offence under this section shall be liable on summary conviction to a fine not exceeding level five on the standard scale.

Monopolies and competition

Competition and anti-competitive practices.
33. – (1) In this section "regulatory provision" means –

(a) any rule made by the General Council;

(b) any provision of the Code of Practice issued by the Council under section 19; and

(c) any other advice or guidance given by the Council, any of its committees or any sub-committee of such a committee.

(2) Schedule 8 to the [1973 c. 41.] Fair Trading Act 1973 (powers exercisable when making certain orders) shall, for the purposes of a competition order, have effect in relation to a regulatory provision as it has effect in relation to an agreement, but with the necessary modifications.

(3) A competition order may be made so as to have effect in relation to a regulatory provision even though that provision was properly made in exercise of functions conferred by this Act.

(4) In this section "a competition order" means –

(a) an order under section 56 of the Act of 1973 (orders following reports on monopoly references); or

(b) an order under section 10 of the [1980 c. 21.] Competition Act 1980 (orders following reports on competition references).

(5) For the purposes of any order under section 56 of the Act of 1973 or section 10 of the Act of 1980, section 90(4) of the Act of 1973 (power to apply orders to existing agreements) shall have effect in relation to a regulatory provision as it has effect in relation to an agreement.

Miscellaneous

Default powers of the Privy Council.

34. – (1) If it appears to the Privy Council that the General Council has failed to perform any functions which, in the opinion of the Privy Council, should have been performed, the Privy Council may give the General Council such direction as the Privy Council considers appropriate.

(2) If the General Council fails to comply with any direction given under this section, the Privy Council may itself give effect to the direction.

(3) For the purpose of enabling it to give effect to a direction under subsection (1), the Privy Council may –

(a) exercise any power of the General Council or do any act or other thing authorised to be done by the General Council; and

(b) do, of its own motion, any act or other thing which it is otherwise authorised to do under this Act on the instigation of the General Council.

Rules.

35. – (1) The approval of the Privy Council shall be required for any exercise by the General Council of a power to make rules under this Act.

(2) Any rules made by the General Council or by Order in Council under this Act may make different provision with respect to different cases, or classes of case and, in particular, different provision with respect to different categories of osteopath or registered osteopath.

(3) Any Order in Council made under section 10(8)(b) or 31(5) shall be subject to annulment in pursuance of a resolution of either House of Parliament.

(4) Nothing in any rules made under this Act shall be taken to oblige or entitle any person to act in breach of the law relating to confidentiality.

Exercise of powers of Privy Council.

36. – (1) Where the approval of the Privy Council is required by this Act in respect of the making of any rules by the General Council, it shall be given by an order made by the Privy Council.

(2) Any power of the Privy Council under this Act to make an order shall be exercisable by statutory instrument.

(3) Any order approving rules made under section 5, 8(8), 17 or 30 shall be subject to annulment in pursuance of a resolution of either House of Parliament.

(4) For the purposes of exercising any powers conferred by this Act (other than the power of hearing appeals) the quorum of the Privy Council shall be two.

(5) Any act of the Privy Council under this Act shall be sufficiently signified by an instrument signed by the Clerk of the Council.

(6) Any document purporting to be –

(a) an instrument made by the Privy Council under this Act, and

(b) signed by the Clerk of the Privy Council,

shall be evidence (and in Scotland sufficient evidence) of the fact that the instrument was so made and of its terms.

Professional indemnity insurance.

37. – (1) The General Council may by rules make provision requiring –

(a) registered osteopaths who are practising as osteopaths, or

(b) prescribed categories of registered osteopaths who are practising as osteopaths,

to secure that they are properly insured against liability to, or in relation to, their patients.

(2) The rules may, in particular –

(a) prescribe risks, or descriptions of risk, with respect to which insurance is required;

(b) prescribe the amount of insurance that is required either generally or with respect to prescribed risks;

(c) make such provision as the General Council considers appropriate for the purpose of securing, so far as is reasonably practicable, that the requirements of the rules are complied with;

(d) make provision with respect to failure to comply with their requirements (including provision for treating any failure as constituting unacceptable professional conduct).

Data protection and access to personal health information.

38. – (1) In section 2(1) of the [1990 c. 23.] Access to Health Records Act 1990 (definition of health professionals), after paragraph (f) there shall be inserted –

"(ff) a registered osteopath;"

(2) The following instruments shall be amended as mentioned in subsection (3) –

(a) the [S.I. 1987/1903.] Data Protection (Subject Access Modification) (Health) Order 1987;

(b) the [S.I. 1989/206.] Access to Personal Files (Social Services) Regulations 1989;

(c) the [S.I. 1989/251.] Access to Personal Files (Social Work) (Scotland) Regulations 1989;

(d) the [S.I. 1989/503.] Access to Personal Files (Housing) Regulations 1989; and

(e) the [S.I. 1992/1852.] Access to Personal Files (Housing) (Scotland) Regulations 1992.

(3) In each case, at the end of the Table in the Schedule there shall be inserted –

"

Registered osteopath   Osteopaths Act 1993, section 41.
"

(4) The reference in section 2(1) of the [1988 c. 28.] Access to

Medical Reports Act 1988 to the order mentioned in subsection (2)(a) shall be read as a reference to that order as amended by this section.

(5) The amendments made by this section shall not be taken to prejudice the power to make further orders or (as the case may be) regulations varying or revoking the amended provisions.

Exemption from provisions about rehabilitation of offenders.

39. – (1) In this section –

"the 1975 Order" means the [S.I. 1975/1023.] Rehabilitation of Offenders Act 1974 (Exceptions) Order 1975 (professions etc. with respect to which provisions of the Act of 1974 are excluded); and

"the 1979 Order" means the [S.R. 1979 No. 195.] Rehabilitation of Offenders (Exceptions) Order (Northern Ireland) 1979 (professions etc. with respect to which provisions of the [S.I. 1978/1908 (N.I. 27).] Rehabilitation of Offenders (Northern Ireland) Order 1978 are excluded).

(2) In Part I of Schedule 1 to the 1975 Order, there shall be inserted at the end –

" 11. Registered osteopath."

(3) In Part I of Schedule 1 to the 1979 Order, there shall be inserted at the end –

" 10. Registered osteopath."

(4) In both the 1975 Order and the 1979 Order, in each case in Part IV of Schedule 1, there shall be inserted in the appropriate place –

" "registered osteopath" has the meaning given by section 41 of the Osteopaths Act 1993."

(5) The amendment of the 1975 Order and the 1979 Order by this section shall not be taken to prejudice the power to make further orders varying or revoking the amended provisions.

Financial provisions.

40. – (1) The General Council shall keep proper accounts of all sums received or paid by it and proper records in relation to those accounts.

(2) The accounts for each financial year of the General Council shall be audited by persons appointed by the Council.

(3) No person may be appointed as an auditor under subsection (2) unless he is eligible for appointment as a company auditor under section 25 of the [1989 c. 40.] Companies Act 1989 or Article 28 of the [S.I. 1990/593 (N.I. 5).] Companies (Northern Ireland) Order 1990.

(4) As soon as is reasonably practicable after the accounts of the General Council have been audited, the Council shall –

(a) cause them to be published, together with any report on them made by the auditors; and

(b) send a copy of the accounts and of any such report to the Privy Council.

(5) The Privy Council shall lay any copy sent to them under subsection (4) before each House of Parliament.

Supplemental

Interpretation.   **41.** In this Act –

"conditionally registered osteopath" means a person who is registered with conditional registration;

"fully registered osteopath" means a person who is registered with full registration;

"the General Council" means the General Osteopathic Council;

"interim suspension order" has the meaning given in section 24(3);

"opening of the register" means the date on which section 3 comes into force;

"prescribed" means prescribed by rules made by the General Council;

"provisionally registered osteopath" means a person who is registered with provisional registration;

"recognised qualification" has the meaning given by section 14(1);

"the register" means the register of osteopaths maintained by the Registrar under section 2;

"registered" means registered in the register;

"registered address", in relation to a registered osteopath, means the address which is entered in the register;

"registered osteopath" means a person who is registered as a fully registered osteopath, as a conditionally registered osteopath or as a provisionally registered osteopath;

"the Registrar" has the meaning given in section 2(2);

"the required standard of proficiency" means the standard determined by the General Council under section 13;

"the statutory committees" has the meaning given by section 1(6);

"unacceptable professional conduct" has the meaning given by section 20(2);

"visitor" means a person appointed under section 12.

Short title, commencement, transitional provisions and extent.

42. – (1) This Act may be cited as the Osteopaths Act 1993.

(2) This Act shall come into force on such day as the Secretary of State may by order appoint.

(3) The power conferred by subsection (2) shall be exercisable by statutory instrument.

(4) Different days may be appointed by an order under subsection (2) for different purposes and different provisions.

(5) Any order under subsection (2) may make such transitional provision as the Secretary of State considers appropriate.

(6) The transitional provisions of Part III of the Schedule shall have effect.

(7) This Act extends to the United Kingdom except that –

(a) section 38(1) and section 39(2) extend only to Great Britain;

(b) section 38(2)(c) and (e) extends only to Scotland;

(c) section 39(3) extends only to Northern Ireland; and

(d) section 38(2)(b) and (d) extend only to England and Wales.

INDEX

T - #0656 - 101024 - C0 - 246/174/12 - PB - 9781857757378 - Gloss Lamination